SMOKING AND TOBACCO USE

NEW RESEARCH ON TOBACCO

SMOKING AND TOBACCO USE

Additional books and e-books in this series can be found on Nova's website under the Series tab.

SMOKING AND TOBACCO USE

NEW RESEARCH ON TOBACCO

UTA DREHER
EDITOR

nova
Medicine & Health
New York

Library of Congress Cataloging-in-Publication Data

Names: Dreher, Uta, editor.
Title: New Research on Tobacco
Description: New York: Nova Science Publishers, [2019] | Series: Smoking and Tobacco Use | Includes bibliographical references and index.
Identifiers: LCCN 2019957638 (print) | ISBN 9781536170771 (paperback) |
ISBN 9781536172287 (adobe pdf)

Published by Nova Science Publishers, Inc. † New York

CONTENTS

PREFACE

New Research on Tobacco summarizes the history of tobacco, providing an overview of the markets, the available products, and manufacturing processes. The authors discuss the current regulatory environment within the U.S., as well as the efforts being made by the Food and Drug Administration to reduce the harm that tobacco products inflict on society.

The important discoveries in tobacco research are addressed, and researchers and scientists are encouraged to continue using tobacco as a research tool due to the wealth of existing scientific information about it.

The penultimate chapter focuses on electronic nicotine delivery system, also known as vapes, mods, or e-cigarettes, which have become popular over the years. They have tapped into a billion dollar industry and appear to be staying for good in an ever increasing market.

The concluding study examines tobacco consumption in India. The findings reveal that the respondents living in rural areas consumed more tobacco than those in urban spaces.

Chapter 1 - The tobacco plant is native to North and South America but spread rapidly throughout the world in the 16th century by seafarers. Since then, various forms of tobacco usage have captivated a substantial proportion of the human population. Although cigarettes sales in most industrial countries are declining, the health consequences associated with tobacco usage still takes an enormous toll, accounting for more than 480,000 deaths per year in the U.S. alone. Manufacturing industries currently produce a variety of tobacco products, such as cigarettes, cigars, cigarillos, bidis, kreteks, dissolvables, nicotine patches, nicotine gels, chewable gums, smokeless tobacco products, electronic cigarettes and water pipes. The unifying property of these diverse products is that they all contain nicotine. This enigmatic compound is the primary addictive component of all tobacco products, but it is not a carcinogen. The array of tobacco products currently available differ substantially in their propensity to produce and transfer toxic compounds to the user. Combustible products such as cigarettes are considered to be the most harmful, as the majority of the characterized toxicants found in the smoke have been shown to be products of combustion. Concomitant with the recent introduction of new classes of noncombustible tobacco products (like vaping and heat-not-burned products), are questions faced by regulatory agencies with respect to how these should be regulated and taxed in comparison to their combusted counterparts. In this chapter, the authors summarize the history of tobacco, provide an overview of the markets, the available products, and manufacturing processes. Finally, the authors discuss the currently regulatory environment within the U.S. and the efforts being made by the Food and Drug Administration to reduce the harm that tobacco products inflict on society.

Chapter 2 - Cultivated tobacco (*Nicotiana tabacum* L.) indigenous to North and South America, is the most widely grown commercial non-food cash crop across the world. The characteristic and unique features of tobacco plant include its leaf as commercial-value, short-duration, ability to grow quickly on soils even unsuitable for other crops, relatively resistant to insect-pests attack, relatively easy to harvest, yields millions of seeds/plant and readily amenable to the good agricultural practices. Owing to characteristic nicotine content, tobacco leaves are commercially grown and processed into various tobacco products. Conventionally, tobacco is used in the manufacture of various 'smoke' and 'smokeless' products. Most of the scientific literature on tobacco is also devoted to industrial cigarettes manufacturing. Nevertheless in recent times, tobacco as an alternate source for various food and personal care products, paper industries, biofuel etc. has been exploited. Apart from this, tobacco plant has been also used as an excellent model for biological research in gaining fundamental knowledge in diverse areas of plant-biology. Over the past few decades, major pioneering investigations in plant-science *viz.* genetic-engineering, transgenic research, post-harvest technology, tissue-culture, nutrition and plant-growth, genetics, plant-breeding, photosynthesis, photo-periodism, biochemistry, cytology, molecular-biology, molecular-genetics, parasexual-hybridization, polyploidization, evolutionary-biology, phylogenetic, phytopathology, virology, genomics, choloroplast-genomics, epigenetics, organic-metabolism, molecular-pharming and others areas as well, owe their inception to experimentation with tobacco plants. Besides, tobacco has an incredible history to utilize as an efficient bio-factory for the valuable source of numerous phytochemicals with agricultural, pharmaceuticals and industrial applications. Realizing the enormous potential of tobacco to the mankind, this chapter is a comprehensive overview of tobacco and its application in basic and applied sciences. The purpose of this chapter is to compile and cherish the important discoveries in tobacco research and encourage researchers and scientists to continue using tobacco as a research tool because of wealth of existing scientific information about it and great potential for yet so unexplored benefits and application.

Chapter 3 - Electronic nicotine delivery system (ENDS), also known as vapes, mods, or e-cigarettes, have become popular over the years. They have tapped into a billion dollar industry, and appear to be staying for good in an ever increasing market. Once touted as a tobacco cessation tool, ENDS have created a sub-niche with many flavors, customizations, and lobbying groups. ENDS, in users eyes, do not hold the stigma associated with combustible tobacco cigarettes. They are perceived as a socially acceptable, healthier alternative that lacks the health detriments of traditional tobacco products. Their target market is not only adults, but also minors, with common flavors such as bubble gum, vanilla, and watermelon. Surveys of young teens have shown that the percentage of minors using ENDS is growing, year over year. The ENDS products themselves also offer different customizations, ranging from longer lasting batteries to larger reservoirs. In regards to regulation, the US Food and Drug Administration (FDA) recently extended its authority over tobacco products to include ENDS. One such change brought on by the

FDA are box labels to warn of nicotine addiction on ENDS products, similar to their combustible counterparts.

Chapter 4 - This study examines the early and late age at initiation of tobacco consumption in India. It uses Global Adult Tobacco Survey (2009-10) data to this end. Bivariate and multivariate statistical techniques are used to analyze the data set. The findings reveal that the respondents living in rural areas were highly initiated in different forms of tobacco as compared with urban space. Education was one of the primary factors for initiation of tobacco use. Respondents having secondary and above education were highly initiated in late age. However, the age of tobacco initiation either early or late was significantly higher (7 per cent) among males as compared with females. Respondents belonging to the central (4.9 per cent) and northern regions (4.6 per cent) were highly initiated to tobacco as compared with other regions. Considering a decline in the initiation of tobacco consumption, local level awareness and catchy programmes play an effective role. In this, the involvement of children, women and leaders can be help to reach the goal.

In: New Research on Tobacco
Editor: Uta Dreher
ISBN: 978-1-53617-077-1

Chapter 1

TOBACCO: PAST, PRESENT, AND FUTURE

Niharika Nonavinakere Chandrakanth*
and Ralph E. Dewey
Dept. of Crop and Soil Sciences,
North Carolina State University, Raleigh, NC US

ABSTRACT

The tobacco plant is native to North and South America but spread rapidly throughout the world in the 16th century by seafarers. Since then, various forms of tobacco usage have captivated a substantial proportion of the human population. Although cigarettes sales in most industrial countries are declining, the health consequences associated with tobacco usage still takes an enormous toll, accounting for more than 480,000 deaths per year in the U.S. alone. Manufacturing industries currently produce a variety of tobacco products, such as cigarettes, cigars, cigarillos, bidis, kreteks, dissolvables, nicotine patches, nicotine gels, chewable gums, smokeless tobacco products, electronic cigarettes and water pipes. The unifying property of these diverse products is that they all contain nicotine. This enigmatic compound is the primary addictive component of all tobacco products, but it is not a carcinogen. The array of tobacco products

---

* Corresponding Author's Email: nnonavi@ncsu.edu.

currently available differ substantially in their propensity to produce and transfer toxic compounds to the user. Combustible products such as cigarettes are considered to be the most harmful, as the majority of the characterized toxicants found in the smoke have been shown to be products of combustion. Concomitant with the recent introduction of new classes of noncombustible tobacco products (like vaping and heat-not-burned products), are questions faced by regulatory agencies with respect to how these should be regulated and taxed in comparison to their combusted counterparts. In this chapter, we summarize the history of tobacco, provide an overview of the markets, the available products, and manufacturing processes. Finally, we discuss the currently regulatory environment within the U.S. and the efforts being made by the Food and Drug Administration to reduce the harm that tobacco products inflict on society.

Keywords: history of tobacco, tobacco products, tobacco market, FDA regulations on tobacco products

1. History of Tobacco

Christopher Columbus wrote about receiving pungent dried leaves as a gift from the Native Americans in his journal. The leaves were thrown away, but later Columbus found that they were considered to be of high value. Tobacco is native to the Americas, and the indigenous populations typically consumed crude aqueous extracts or chewed on green leaves. The smoking of tobacco was innovated by two Europeans, Rodrigo de Jerez and Luis Torres. Rodrigo de Jerez is known as the first European smoker. In the 16th century, as sea routes became established, there was a rapid spread of tobacco seeds by sailors. Tobacco was introduced in Portugal, Spain, Japan, France, Turkey, and England, among others. Tobacco was initially utilized as a medicine and was even compulsory for a time at the elite Eton College, as people believed that it helped ward off infections. Published in Antwerp, Belgium in the 1580s, "De herbe panacea" was the first known work entirely dedicated to tobacco, describing various tobacco recipes and claims that it could cure diseases. Around the same time, a German writer gave the first recorded caution about using tobacco by calling it a "violent herb." [1].

In terms of tobacco usage, the 17th century could aptly be referred to as the age of pipes, due to the rising popularity of pipes as the means of consumption. During this period, large-scale cultivation of tobacco expanded across many regions of North and South America. In places such as Virginia, tobacco was even used as currency. In 1753, Carolus Linnaeus designated the genus of tobacco as *Nicotiana*, with the initial two recognized species being *Nicotiana rustica* and *Nicotiana tabacum*. Suspicions concerning negative health consequences also began to appear, as John Hill from England reported in 1761 that the excessive use of snuff made people vulnerable to nose cancer [1].

The 19th and 20th centuries could be called the age of cigarettes, as this form of consumption grew to predominate [1, 2]. In the early 1800's Gaspare Cerioli and Louis Vanquelin (independently) isolated nicotine from smoke, which was called the essence of tobacco. Later, Wilhelm Heinrich Posselt and Karl Ludwig Reimann purified nicotine directly from the tobacco plant. In 1889, Langley and Dickinson conducted revolutionary studies on the effects of nicotine on the ganglia. A. Pictet and P. Crepieux first synthesized pure nicotine in 1893. In 1965, the Federal Cigarette Labeling and Advertising Act required that the Surgeon General's warning, "Caution: Cigarette Smoking May Be Hazardous to Your Health," the first of what would become many warning labels, be placed on each cigarette package.

Recent landmarks include the discovery and marketing of the nicotine patch and nicotine gums in the mid-1980s, products that have been utilized by millions of people to help them quit smoking [3]. In 2003, electronic cigarettes were first commercialized [4]. Currently, a broad array of tobacco and tobacco-derived products are available to consumers; for example, cigarettes, cigars, little cigars, cigarillos, bidis, kreteks (containing cloves), dissolvable products, nicotine patches, chewable gums, various smokeless tobacco products, electronic cigarettes, and water pipes [5].

2. Tobacco Markets

2.1. Global Tobacco Market

The giants of the global tobacco industry include Philip Morris International (PMI), British American Tobacco (BAT), Imperial Tobacco Company, Altria Group, Reynolds American, Hongyunhonghe Tobacco, Japan Tobacco, Gudang Garam Tobacco, and Korea Tobacco and Ginseng Corporation. In 2018, PMI was ranked number one worldwide, based on net sales [6, 7]·

Currently, cigarettes command the largest share of the global tobacco market. According to Grand View Research, Inc., the global tobacco market size is expected to reach approximately US $700 billion by 2021, with a 2.8% compound annual growth rate (CAGR) from 2016 to 2021 [6]. Recent estimates by BAT, however, placed the current global tobacco market as being worth approximately US $760 billion. It is important to note that these estimates exclude China, the world's largest producer and consumer of tobacco products. Of BAT's estimated global market valuation of US $760, US $680 billion is attributed to the sale of conventional cigarettes. In 2016, the global sales of what has been termed Next Generation Products (NGPs) like e-cigarettes, vaping and heat-not-burned (HNB) accounted for approximately US $12.3 billion. The market share of NGPs is expected to increase substantially in the future [8].

2.2. US Tobacco Market

According to an Ibis World report on the US cigarette and tobacco manufacturing industry, cigarette sales have been declining in recent years due to a decrease in the number of smokers, rising public scrutiny, stringent regulations, and increased excise taxes. The tobacco industries in the US are thus focusing on developing alternative products like e-cigarettes that have lower health risks. Increased demand for e-cigarettes and other noncombustible tobacco products are balancing some of the decrease in sales of traditional cigarettes [9]. In the US, cigarette and tobacco manufacturing generates approximately $46.3 billion annually. Traditional cigarettes account for 70.7% of that revenue. E-vapor products, smokeless tobacco, cigars and other products like pipe tobacco, and alternative products such as clove cigarettes, homogenized and reconstituted tobacco, tobacco extracts and essences accounts for 13.8%, 9.8%, 1.8%, and 3.9%, respectively [9].

The biggest participants in the US cigarette and tobacco manufacturing industry include Altria Group, Reynolds American, Imperial brands, Vector Group and others, accounting for 54.4%, 28.5%, 8.1%, 2.4%, and 6.6% of the market share, respectively [9]. In 2003, Philip Morris Companies Inc. changed its name to Altria Group. The Altria family of companies includes Philip Morris USA, US Smokeless Tobacco Company, John Middleton (cigars), Nat Sherman, Nu Mark (an innovation company that makes e-vapor product), Ste. Michelle Wine Estates, and Philip Morris Capital Corporation [10]. Recently, Altria acquired a 35% stake in Juul Labs, which is the most popular e-cigarette brand in the United States [9]. Ibis World predicts that US cigarette and tobacco manufacturing industry annual revenues will decrease to $44.2 billion by 2023 [9].

3. Tobacco Products

Tobacco products can be broadly divided into three categories: (1) combustible tobacco products; (2) smokeless tobacco products; (3) and E-vapor products.

3.1. Combustible Tobacco Products

Tobacco products that require combustion during use include cigarettes, cigars, cigarillos, roll your own tobacco, pipe tobacco, and other minor products. Cigarettes are defined as any form of tobacco that is wrapped in a paper or substance that is not made from tobacco. Small cigarettes are defined as cigarettes weighing no more than three pounds per thousand, and large cigarettes are those weighing more than three pounds per thousand [11]. It has been estimated that currently around 5,500 billion cigarettes are being consumed in the US each year [7]. Popular cigarette brands in the US include Marlboro, Newport, Camel, Pall Mall, Maverick, Santa Fe, Winston and Kool. Based on 2017 sales data, Marlboro (Altria Group) was the leading brand, followed by Newport and Camel (Reynolds American) [12]. Cigarettes are often flavored with menthol and other flavoring agents to reduce the harshness, bitterness, and astringency of the tobacco smoke. The 2009 Family Smoking Prevention and Tobacco Control Act, however, banned the sale of cigarettes with flavors other than menthol.

Cigars are any roll of tobacco wrapped in leaf tobacco or other matrix containing tobacco. Similar to the classification of cigarettes, small cigars are defined as those that weigh less than three pounds per thousand, with large cigars being those that weigh more than three pounds per thousand [11]. Based on 2015 sales data, Swisher little (a small cigar type) was the leading cigar brand in the US. Swisher little was followed by Swisher sweets (large cigars and cigarillos) and Black & Mild (large cigars and cigarillos) [12]. Cigarillos are small and narrow cigars that fundamentally differ from cigarettes in that they are wrapped in tobacco leaf, as opposed to paper [9]. Roll your own tobaccos are the loose tobacco filler used by consumers who prefer to hand roll their cigarettes. Hand-rolled cigarettes are less expensive and are often called rollies, roll-ups, burns, and rolls [13]. Finally, pipe tobacco is loose tobacco designed to be smoked out of a pipe, a once popular form of tobacco usage that now represents a very small portion of the market.

Nicotine is the agent that causes people to become addicted to smoking cigarettes. However, nicotine is not a direct chemical carcinogen. Tobacco smoke contains more than 7,000 chemicals, of which at least 69 of these have been associated with causing cancer [14]. In addition to carcinogens, other classes of toxicants are also present in tobacco smoke that contribute to different smoking-related pathologies. Among the more notable harmful and potentially harmful chemicals (HPHCs) found in tobacco smoke are lead, cadmium, acrolein, acetaldehyde, benzene, ammonia, carbon monoxide, 1,3-butadiene, tobacco-specific nitrosamines (TSNAs), and polycyclic aromatic hydrocarbons. The FDA has listed 93 known HPHCs present in tobacco smoke on their website [15].

Tar is the term used to collectively describe the chemical substances produced when tobacco is burned [16]. In addition to the compounds listed above, studies have shown that the tars in cigarette smoke contain free radicals that damage DNA [17]. When tobacco smoke is inhaled, the tar can form a sticky layer on the inside of the lungs. Continued exposure to cigarette smoke may lead to lung cancer, emphysema, or non-lung related problems such as heart disease. Depending on how the cigarettes are made, different amounts of tar are produced [16].

In the 1950s, the use of cigarette filters was initiated in an attempt to trap harmful tar residues. Tobacco companies started manufacturing cigarettes with filters and advertised them as high tar, mild tar, low tar, and ultra-low tar cigarettes. In the US, the 2009 Family Smoking Prevention and Tobacco Control Act prohibited companies from advertising cigarettes as "light," "low," or "mild." This was done to prevent smokers from believing that low or mild cigarettes are less harmful than standard cigarettes [18, 19].

Mainstream smoke is the tobacco smoke directly inhaled by the smoker and exhaled into the environment. Sidestream smoke is the smoke that is released from the burning end of a cigarette, cigar or pipe. Sidestream smoke is inherently more dangerous as it contains higher concentrations of toxic carcinogens than mainstream smoke. The particles in the sidestream smoke are smaller in size and are easily absorbed by cells. Secondhand smoke (SHS), which is also referred to as environmental tobacco smoke, is a mixture of the mainstream smoke exhaled by the smoker into the environment and the sidestream smoke. Passive or involuntary smoking are the terms used when non-smokers are exposed to SHS. SHS contains the same amount of HPHCs as the mainstream smoke inhaled by smokers. SHS can cause lung cancer, even if the person has never smoked [20, 21, 22]. Hence, most governments worldwide have banned smoking in public places.

3.2. Smokeless Tobacco Products

Smokeless tobacco products include chewing tobacco, snuff (moist, and dry), snus, and dissolvable tobacco products. Chewing tobacco is cured tobacco packaged in different forms, like loose leaves, plugs (compressed small brick-shaped leaves) and twists (braids of leaves). Chewing tobacco is placed in the mouth between the cheek and gum, and the saliva that builds up is generally spit out or swallowed. Chewing tobacco can also be flavored [23, 24].

Tobacco that is finely cut or ground and packaged in small tins or teabag-like pouches is used as snuff. It is available in both dry and moist forms. A small amount of snuff is placed either along the gum line, behind the lip, or between the gum and the cheek. An act of using snuff is also called dipping. Dry snuff is often sniffed through the nose, and like chewing tobacco can also be flavored [23, 24]. Snus is a flavored tobacco product that originated in Sweden. Snus is like snuff, except that the tobacco is pasteurized during the manufacturing process to kill the bacteria that can produce harmful metabolites, particularly TSNAs [23, 24]. Levi Garrett Plug, Day's work, Red Man, Grizzly, and Copenhagen are some of the leading smokeless tobacco brands [12]. Smokeless tobaccos are often promoted as less harmful products. However, they have still been associated with increased risk of oral cancer, esophageal cancer, pancreatic cancer, stillbirth or perinatal death, and other diseases. [14, 24].

Dissolvable tobacco products are generally flavored and are sold as lozenges, strips, sticks, and orbs/pellets that dissolve in the mouth and do not require spitting out the product. These products look like candies and are marketed for therapeutic purposes such as aids to help people quit smoking. Nicotine gels, patches and gums are noncombustible tobacco products. The nicotine gels and transdermal patches are applied to the skin where the nicotine becomes absorbed and directed to the bloodstream. The nicotine gums release nicotine as they are being chewed. These products are mainly marketed to people who are attempting to quit smoking and are collectively referred to as nicotine replacement therapy (NRT) products [24].

3.3. E – vapor Products

A wide variety of electronic nicotine delivery systems (ENDS) are being manufactured and are termed as vapes, vaporizers, vape pens, hookah pens, electronic cigarettes (e-cigarettes or e-cigs), and e-pipes. These products are noncombustible tobacco products. In the case of ENDS, the e–liquid is heated to create an aerosol, which is inhaled by the user. E-liquids are produced with varying concentrations of nicotine, and can also include flavoring agents, propylene glycol, vegetable glycerin, and other ingredients as described below [9, 24].

A patent granted to Joseph Robinson in 1931 is the first documented reference to an electronic cigarette model. [25]. In 1965, Herbert A. Gilbert from Beaver Falls, PA patented the first smoke-free, non-tobacco cigarette device. Around 1979, Phil Ray with Norman Jacobson created the first commercialized variation of an e-cigarette. However, this device proved to be unsuccessful. Norman Jacobson attributed the failure of the device to be due to an inherently faulty design. Later in the 20th century, RJ Reynolds Tobacco and Philip Morris USA introduced Eclipse and Accord, respectively. Both products were "heat-not-burned" devices, meaning that the tobacco in them is not exposed to temperatures high enough to initiate combustion. Both Eclipse and Accord failed to establish a sizeable consumer base. In 2003, Chinese pharmacist Hon Lik created the first commercially successful e-cigarette. Hon Lik commercialized e-cigarettes in China through the company Golden Dragon Holdings. This company later changed its name to Ruyan meaning "like smoke." In 2006-2007 electronic cigarettes were introduced in Europe and the US [26, 27].

E-cigarette devices contain the following components: a battery, a reservoir for holding an e-liquid (generally containing nicotine), a heating element or an atomizer, and a mouthpiece through which the user inhales. The device heats the e-liquid, also called e- juice, into an aerosol that is inhaled. E-liquid is mainly composed of propylene glycol and/or vegetable glycerin as the solvent for the nicotine. They are most often flavored. According to a study conducted by Zhu et al., in 2014, over 7,500 different flavors had been incorporated into these products. Among the most popular flavors were those tasting like various fruits, candies, mint, coffee, bubble-gum, as well as novel flavors such as Belgium waffle and those mimicking alcoholic drinks. Custom flavors can also be made based on the customer's preference. These flavors are playing a key role in attracting young consumers [28].

The first-generation of e-cigarette devices were designed to look like conventional cigarettes and were often called cigalikes. Some were also manufactured in the shape of cigars and pipes. Newer models were designed with a cartridge to hold the e-liquid, which was either prefilled and disposable, or could be used then refilled by the user. Second-generation devices included pen-shaped products referred to as "tank systems" and are larger in shape. Third- and fourth-generation devices included products with even different shapes, such as USB-like (rectangular), square, or cylindrical. E-cigarette devices can also be built by customers on their own using individual parts and are referred to as "mods." The various e-cigarette brands differ in terms of design, amount of aerosol particles, nicotine content, flavoring agents, and solvents used [28].

In 2016, the global e-cigarette and vaping markets were valued at US $7.19 billion [29]. According to "Research and Market's Report on E-Cigarette Market by Product - Global Size, Share, Development, Growth, and Demand Forecast, 2013-2023", the e-cigarette market is estimated to reach $44.6 billion by 2023. The US is currently the largest e-cigarette market, followed by the UK and China [30]. E-cigarette product manufacture, however, is largely localized in Shenzhen, Guangdong Province, China [28].

The major industry players in the e-cigarette market include: BAT, Altria Group, Japan Tobacco, Imperial Brands, PMI, VMR Products, NJOY Inc, International Vapor Group, Vapor Hub International, and FIN Branding Group [30]. Altria owns the brands MarkTen and Green Smoke. Recently, Altria purchased a 35% stake in e-cigarette maker Juul, worth $12.8 billion [32]. Juul represented more than two-thirds of the e-cigarette market at the time of this purchase [31]. VUSE (R. J. Reynolds Vapor Company), Puritane (Formerly Ruyan, later acquired by Imperial Tobacco), blu (Lorillard Vapor Company until 2015, later acquired by Imperial Tobacco), VYPE (BAT), E-

Swisher (Swisher), E-lites, and Ploom (Japan Tobacco International) are other popular e-cigarette brands [28]. E-cigarettes are available for sale in convenience stores, tobacco stores, pharmacies, Costco (and other countrywide chains), online retailers, and shops dedicated to e-cigarette products called "vape shops". E-cigarettes can also be used as marijuana delivery systems. Ploom PAX (Japan Tobacco International) is one such product [28].

PMI has been the leader in the resurgence of heat-not-burned tobacco products. IQOS is the name of their first and most successful heat-not-burned commercialized product. PMI has claimed that 6.6 million smokers have quit smoking conventional cigarettes and switched to IQOS. IQOS heats the tobacco to comparatively low temperatures (up to 350°C), sufficiently high to release nicotine and aromatic components associated with flavor, but without producing combustion, fire, ash, or smoke. In contrast, traditional cigarettes burn at temperatures over 600°C, generating a plethora of harmful chemicals that are the products of combustion. As the tobacco in IQOS is merely heated and not burned, the levels of harmful chemicals are significantly reduced. TEEPS is another PMI product, similar to IQOS but using an alternative heating source. In 2014, PMI acquired Nicocigs, a leading e-cigarette company in the UK that produces disposables, rechargeables, and tank systems. Also, Altria Group has made its e-cigarette products available to PMI for commercialization outside the US. PMI's next generation e-vapor product is called IQOS MESH. Another product called STEEM is still under development. STEEM generates a nicotine-containing vapor in the form of a nicotine salt which can be more easily inhaled by the consumer [33].

E-cigarettes, and more recently heat-not-burned products, are manufactured as a better alternative to conventional cigarettes. E-cigarettes produce fewer harmful chemicals when compared to traditional tobacco smoke. Even toxicants that are found in the unburned tobacco tend to be greatly reduced in e-cigarettes and other vaping products. TSNAs, for example, are potent carcinogenic agents generated primarily during the curing of the tobacco leaves and are thus present in cigarettes prior to combustion. These compounds are filtered during the manufacturing of the e-liquids, however, and studies have shown that the e-liquid and its corresponding aerosol contain only minimal amounts of TSNAs [34, 35, 36].

E-cigarettes have both advantages and disadvantages. Their usage is clearly advantageous to existing adult smokers. In addition to reducing toxicant exposure, switching to e-cigarettes may also help adult smokers quit smoking. However, definitive data in this regard is still lacking. E-cigarettes are not considered safe for children, young adults, pregnant woman, and for first-time users of tobacco products. Unfortunately, youth have become highly attracted to e-cigarettes. The flavoring agents in the e-liquid play a key role in attracting young users. In 2018, approximately 3.6 million US middle school (4.9%) and high school students (20.8%) reported using e-cigarettes [36]. As a result, the FDA is currently considering the implementation of regulations that would ban or severely restrict the addition of flavorings in vaping products, or at least the sale of these products in stores accessible to minors.

4. Tobacco Varieties and Cigarette Blends

Tobacco plants are transplanted to the field when they are around 15-20 cm high. It takes roughly two months for a tobacco seed to grow into a plant of this height. After transplant, the tobacco plants are grown in the field for another two to three months and are harvested differently based on the plant variety. The three main tobacco types used in cigarette manufacturing are Virginia, burley and oriental. These varieties are grown in over thirty countries including Argentina, Brazil, China, and the United States. Virginia and oriental tobaccos are harvested leaf by leaf, whereas the whole plant is harvested in the case of burley tobaccos. An additional market type known as dark tobaccos is used in the production of smokeless tobacco products [37].

Curing is the next major step post-harvest. It refers to the drying of the mature leaf and largely defines the character and ultimate leaf quality. The curing processes differ depending on the variety and the desired end product. For example, cigarettes produced according to what is referred to as the

"American Blend" are made using a combination of the three major tobacco types. For this blend the burley tobacco is air-cured, the Virginia tobacco is flue-cured, and the oriental plants are sun-cured. In the case of flue-curing, the leaves are hung in a barn and heated air is circulated to dry the leaves. Air-curing involves hanging the leaves in a well-ventilated barn and allowing them to dry for up to eight weeks. Finally, sun-curing refers to exposing the leaves to the sun for about two weeks. In each case, the leaves gradually lose moisture and develop a distinct aroma, texture, and color [37].

After curing the leaves are typically sorted by stalk position and quality grade. The sorted leaves are then packed in bales for evaluation by leaf buyers. The leaves are separated from the stem in the case of burley and Virginia tobaccos. Finally, the leaves undergo processing to remove sand and non-tobacco matter. The processed, dried leaves are then blended and incorporated into cigarettes. Sugars like sucrose are sometimes added to make up for the sugars lost during the curing process; other ingredients that impact flavor such as menthol can also be added [37].

Virginia tobacco is also known as bright tobacco as it turns golden-yellow to deep orange during curing. Burley tobacco is generally light to dark brown after curing. Oriental tobaccos are best known for their highly aromatic properties. The two most commonly used cigarettes blends are the American Blend (mentioned above) that combines portions of all three tobacco types, and the Virginia Blend, which is produced only using Virginia style tobaccos. American blend cigarettes predominate the markets in the US, Japan, most of Europe, South America and Africa. Virginia blend cigarettes are the most popular cigarette type in the UK, Canada, Australia and China [37].

5. Regulation of Tobacco Products

Globally, approximately 5.4 million people die due to tobacco-related illnesses every year. The death rate is expected to increase to more than 8 million/year by 2030 [38]. Among adults in the US, cigarette smoking has declined from 42% in 1965 to 18% in 2012 [14]. In spite of this decrease, nearly 40 million US adults still smoke cigarettes. In 2018, about 4.7 million middle and high school students were reported to use at least one form of tobacco product, 3.6 million of whom were e-cigarette users. In the US, cigarette smoking is responsible for more than 480,000 deaths per year. This includes more than 41,000 deaths resulting from SHS exposure. Smoking is responsible for more deaths each year than the total number of deaths caused by HIV, illegal drug use, alcohol use, motor vehicle injuries, and firearm-related incidents combined. About 90% of all lung cancer deaths are caused by smoking tobacco. The negative effects of tobacco cost approximately $300 billion every year, of which nearly $170 billion is spent on medical care to treat smoking-related disease in adults, and more than $156 billion in lost productivity due to premature death and exposure to SHS [39]. On average, it has been estimated that every cigarette takes 11 minutes off the smoker's life [40].

To reduce the adverse effects of tobacco and to create a healthier future for Americans, on June 22, 2009, President Obama signed the Family Smoking Prevention and Tobacco Control Act into law. This law granted the FDA authority to regulate the manufacture, import, packaging, labeling, advertising, promotion, sale, and distribution of cigarettes, roll your own tobacco, the tobacco rolling paper, and smokeless tobacco products like chewable tobaccos, snus and some dissolvables [19, 41, 42]. In 2016, the FDA extended their regulatory authority to include cigars, pipe tobacco, all dissolvables, nicotine gels, hookah tobacco, electronic nicotine delivery systems (ENDS) and their components. Dissolvables and nicotine gels are marketed for therapeutic purposes and are regulated by the FDA through the Center for Drug Evaluation and Research (CDER) as drugs.

The 2009 Tobacco Control Act restricted tobacco marketing and sales to youth, and mandated warning labels on smokeless tobacco products. Smokeless tobacco packaging must contain at least one of the following warning labels: "this product can cause mouth cancer"; "this product can cause gum disease and tooth loss"; "this product is not a safe alternative to cigarettes"; or "smokeless tobacco is addictive". These warnings were aimed to increase the awareness of the health risks associated with smokeless tobacco. With respect to cigarettes, the Tobacco Control Act prohibited tobacco companies from making reduced harm claims like "light," "low," or "mild," without having first applied for and received approval of the product being officially designated as a modified risk tobacco product. This step was taken to prevent the consumers to falsely believe that products labeled "light," "low," or "mild," are safer than regular cigarettes. The Tobacco Control Act mandated that tobacco companies provide the FDA with detailed information about the ingredients in their products. This law also preserved the authority of state, local, and tribal governments to regulate tobacco products in specific respects. What the 2009 Tobacco Control Act cannot do is the following: (1) require a prescription to purchase tobacco products; (2) mandate the reduction of nicotine yields to zero; (3) ban face-to-face sales of a particular category of retail outlets; and (4) ban specific classes of tobacco products [19].

In 1994, Benowitz and Henningfield proposed the idea of reducing the nicotine content in cigarettes over time, with the rationale that this would lead to lowering nicotine dependence. As nicotine is the addictive agent, decreasing its content in cigarettes would arguably make them less addictive. This would theoretically lead to fewer young people becoming addicted adult smokers, and for previously addicted smokers, potentially make the act of quitting easier [43]. The nicotine content in most commercial cigarettes ranges from 10 – 15 mg/cigarette. Smokers systemically absorb 10% of the nicotine on average, i.e., 1–2 mg of nicotine per cigarette. The amount of nicotine required to produce reinforcing effects and to sustain addiction differs from person to person. Thus, it would be difficult for the FDA to decide on a threshold nicotine content in cigarettes that could prevent all new smokers from becoming addicted.

Tobacco harm reduction is the term used to refer to a public health strategy to lower the health risks associated with tobacco. Around more than half of the adult smokers in the US (~22 million) are interested in less harmful tobacco products [44, 45]. In July 2017, the FDA announced a comprehensive plan to lower the health risks associated with tobacco. Pursuing the lowering of nicotine to non-addictive levels in cigarettes was one of the key aspects of this plan [41]. Specifically, the FDA has proposed that future cigarettes be produced that limits the nicotine content to 0.5 mg/g (dry weight) in the cut filler tobacco. Producing tobacco plants that can routinely produce nicotine levels this low will be a challenge. However, scientists have found ways in which the genetics of the plant can be altered to lower overall nicotine content, and thus help in meeting this ambitious goal.

In addition to regulating the allowable levels of nicotine in future tobacco products, the FDA has also been granted the authority to mandate the lowering of specific toxicants that are found in these products. One class of toxicant that has received particular attention is the TSNAs, which unlike most of the carcinogens associated with cigarette smoke are typically not the products of combustion, as they are present in the unburned leaf. As a result, TSNAs have been associated with cancers in users of both cigarettes and smokeless tobacco products. One of the most troublesome TSNAs is called N-nitrosonornicotine (NNN), a carcinogen that has been strongly implicated in cancers of the esophagus, and oral and nasal cavities in both smokers and users of chewing tobaccos and snuff. As its first action in the area of potentially regulating toxicant levels in tobacco products, in January of 2017 the FDA submitted a proposal that would restrict the levels of NNN that can be present in smokeless tobacco products to no greater than 1 μg/gram dry weight. Similar to their low nicotine proposal, achieving levels of NNN that are this low is ambitious, and it will not be easy for the industry to meet this standard. Among the more promising strategies that could be implemented to meet such a standard involves mutating the genes in tobacco that are responsible for producing the nornicotine precursor of NNN.

CONCLUSION

Tobacco is native to the Americas and was spread rapidly to many parts of the world in the 16th century by seafarers. Since then, various forms of tobacco usage have captivated a substantial proportion of the human population. Manufacturing industries currently produce a variety of tobacco products, such as cigarettes, cigars, cigarillos, bidis, kreteks, dissolvables, nicotine patches, nicotine gels, chewable gums, smokeless tobacco products, electronic cigarettes and water pipes. The FDA is now authorized to regulate of all these products under the Tobacco Control Act. Fortunately, cigarette sales in many countries are declining due to the decrease in the number of smokers, rising public scrutiny, stringent regulations, and increased excise taxes. Nevertheless, cigarette smoking is still believed to be responsible for more than 480,000 deaths per year in the US alone. The FDA's mission is to reduce the health risks caused by tobacco. One avenue the FDA is pursuing to achieve this goal is a proposed lowering of the nicotine content in cigarettes to non-addictive levels.

Tobacco combustible products are more harmful than smokeless tobacco products, due to the fact that the majority of the characterized toxicants found in the smoke are the products of combustion. Nicotine is not carcinogenic, but some of the nitrosated derivates of nicotine and other alkaloids, referred to as TSNAs, are carcinogens. E-cigarettes were commercialized as an alternative nicotine delivery system for adult smokers. They contain a minimal amount of TSNAs and other carcinogenic agents and are generally considered to be a far safer alternative source of nicotine for adult smokers. However, e-cigarettes cannot be considered entirely harmless, and concern is growing over the rapid increase in the number of youth and young adults who are using e-cigarettes. The FDA is currently making efforts to regulate the type of flavorings permissible in e-cigarettes and vaping products, as well as limit their access as a means of curbing this trend.

References

[1] "Tobacco Timeline." 2019. *Academic.udayton.edu*. Accessed January 16. http://academic.udayton.edu/health/syllabi/tobacco/history2.htm.

[2] Gorrod, J. W, and Peyton Jacob. 1999. Pharmacological significance of nicotine. *Analytical Determination of Nicotine and Related Compounds and Their Metabolites*. Amsterdam: Elsevier.

[3] Rose, J. 1984. "Transdermal Administration of Nicotine." *Drug and Alcohol Dependence* 13 (3): 209-213. doi:10.1016/0376-8716(84) 90061-9.

[4] "Historical Timeline of Electronic Cigarettes – CASAA." 2019. *CASAA*. Accessed January 16. http://www.casaa.org/historical-timeline-of-electronic-cigarettes/.

[5] "Recognize Tobacco in Its Many Forms". 2019. *U.S. Food and Drug Administration*. Accessed January 17. https://www.fda.gov/consumers/consumer-updates/recognize-tobacco-its-many-forms.

[6] "Tobacco Market Size Worth $694.47 Billion By 2021 | CAGR: 2.8%." 2019. *Grandviewresearch.Com*. Accessed January 18. https://www.grandviewresearch.com/press-release/global-tobacco-market.

[7] "Top Tobacco Companies Worldwide 2018 | Statista." 2019. *Statista*. Accessed January 18. https://www.statista.com/statistics/259204/leading-10-tobacco-companies-worldwide-based-on-net-sales/.

[8] "British American Tobacco - The Global Market". 2019. *Bat. Com*. Accessed January 18. http://www.bat.com/group/sites/UK__9D9KCY.nsf/vwPagesWebLive/DO9DCKFM.

[9] IBISWorld, Inc. 2019. "Ibisworld - Industry Market Research, Reports, And Statistics." *Ibisworld.Com*. Accessed January 18. https://www.ibisworld.com/.

[10] "At-A-Glance". 2019. *Altria.Com*. Accessed January 18. http://www.altria.com/About-altria/our-companies/at-a-glance/Pages/default.aspx.

[11] Gorrod, J. W, and Peyton Jacob. 1999. Determination of nicotine in tobacco, tobacco processing environments and tobacco products. *Analytical Determination of Nicotine and Related Compounds and Their Metabolites*. Amsterdam: Elsevier.

[12] "Tobacco Brand Preferences". 2019. *Centers for Disease Control and Prevention*. Accessed January 19. https://www.cdc.gov/tobacco/data_statistics/fact_sheets/tobacco_industry/brand_preference/.

[13] "Should You Roll Your Own Cigarettes?". 2019. *Verywell Mind*. Accessed January 19. https://www.verywellmind.com/the-health-hazards-of-roll-your- own-cigarettes-2825284.

[14] *The Health Consequences of Smoking-50 Years of Progress: A Report of the Surgeon General.* 2014. US Department of Health and Human Services Atlanta, GA: Department of Health and Human Services, Centers for Disease Control and Prevention, National Center for.

[15] "Chemicals in Cigarettes: From Plant to Product to Puff." 2019. *U.S. Food and Drug Administration.* Accessed January 19. https://www.fda.gov/TobaccoProducts/Labeling/ProductsIngredients Components/ucm535235.htm.

[16] "NCI Dictionary of Cancer Terms". 2019. *National Cancer Institute.* Accessed January 19. https://www.cancer.gov/publications/dictionaries/cancer-terms/def/tobacco-tar.

[17] Pryor, William A., Koni Stone, Lun-Yi Zang, and Eliezer Bermúdez. 1998. "Fractionation of Aqueous Cigarette Tar Extracts: Fractions That Contain the Tar Radical Cause DNA Damage." *Chemical Research in Toxicology* 11 (5): 441-448. doi:10.1021/tx970159y.

[18] "Cigarette Tar Carries the Most Toxins." 2019. *Verywell Mind.* Accessed January 19. https://www.verywellmind.com/tar-in-cigarettes-2824718.

[19] "Overview of the Family Smoking Prevention and Tobacco Control Act". 2019. *U.S. Food and Drug Administration.* Accessed January 19. https://www.fda.gov/TobaccoProducts/Labeling/Rules RegulationsGuidance/ucm246129.htm.

[20] "Health Risks of Secondhand Smoke." 2019. *Cancer.Org.* Accessed January 19. https://www.cancer.org/cancer/cancer-causes/tobacco-and-cancer/secondhand-smoke.html.

[21] "How Mainstream Smoke Can Actually Hurt You." 2019. *Verywell Mind.* Accessed January 19. https://www.verywellmind.com/what-is-mainstream-smoke-2824538.

[22] "These Are the Dangers of Sidestream Smoke". 2019. *Verywell Health.* Accessed January 19. https://www.verywellhealth.com/sidestream-smoke-2248934.

[23] "Health Risks of Smokeless Tobacco". 2019. *Cancer.Org.* Accessed January 19. https://www.cancer.org/cancer/cancer-causes/tobacco-and-cancer/smokeless-tobacco.html.

[24] "Smokeless Tobacco Products, Including Dip, Snuff, Chewing Tobacco". 2019. *U.S. Food and Drug Administration*. Accessed January 19. https://www.fda.gov/TobaccoProducts/Labeling/ProductsIngredientsComponents/ucm482582.htm.

[25] Joseph, Robinson. 1927. "Electrical Vaporizer." *USPTO*. US1775947A.

[26] "The History of E-Cigarettes | Electronic Cigarettes the Past, Present and Future | CE Course | Dentalcare.Com." 2019. *Dentalcare.Com*. Accessed January 20. https://www.dentalcare.com/en-us/professional-education/ce-courses/ce451/the-history-of-e-cigarettes.

[27] "Historical Timeline of Electronic Cigarettes - CASAA". 2019. *CASAA*. Accessed January 20. http://www.casaa.org/historical-timeline-of-electronic-cigarettes.

[28] *E-Cigarette Use Among Youth and Young Adults: A Report of the Surgeon General: A Report of the Surgeon General*. 2016. U.S. Department of Health and Human Services, Public Health Service, Office of the Surgeon General, Rockville, MD.

[29] "E-Cigarette & Vaping Market Size & Share | Industry Report, 2018-2025." 2019. *Grandviewresearch.Com*. Accessed January 20. https://www.grandviewresearch.com/industry-analysis/e-cigarette-vaping-market.

[30] "E-Cigarette Market by Product - Global Size, Share, Development, Growth, and Demand Forecast, 2013-2023." 2019. *Researchandmarkets.Com*. Accessed January 20. https://www.researchandmarkets.com/research/hkxdzs/44%E2%80%946%E2%80%94billion?w=4.

[31] "E-Cigarette Sales Have Surged Immensely in the U.S." 2019. *USnews.com*. Accessed January 20. https://www.usnews.com/news/healthiest-communities/articles/2018-08-02/e-cigarette-sales-have-surged-immensely-in-the-us-cdc-study-shows.

[32] David Goldman, CNN Business. 2019. "As Smoking Falls Out of Favor, Altria Looks Beyond Tobacco". *CNN*. Accessed January 23. https://www.cnn.com/2018/12/19/business/altria-juul/index.html.

[33] "Our Smoke-Free Products". 2019. *Pmi.Com.* Accessed January 23. https://www.pmi.com/smoke-free-products.

[34] Farsalinos, Konstantinos, Gene Gillman, Konstantinos Poulas, and Vassilis Voudris. 2015. "Tobacco-Specific Nitrosamines in Electronic Cigarettes: Comparison Between Liquid and Aerosol Levels". *International Journal of Environmental Research and Public Health* 12 (8): 9046-9053. doi:10.3390/ijerph120809046.

[35] McAuley, T. R., P. K. Hopke, J. Zhao, and S. Babaian. 2012. "Comparison of the Effects of E-Cigarette Vapor and Cigarette Smoke on Indoor Air Quality." *Inhalation Toxicology* 24 (12): 850-857. doi:10.3109/08958378.2012.724728.

[36] "About Electronic Cigarettes (E-Cigarettes)". 2019. *Centers for Disease Control and Prevention.* Accessed January 23. https://www.cdc.gov/tobacco/basic_information/e-cigarettes/about-e-cigarettes.html.

[37] "Tobacco Farming". 2019. *Pmi.Com.* Accessed January 24. https://www.pmi.com/our-business/about-us/products/tobacco-farming-and-curing.

[38] "Global Tobacco Control." 2019. *Centers for Disease Control and Prevention.* Accessed January 24. https://www.cdc.gov/tobacco/global/index.htm.

[39] "Fast Facts." 2019. *Centers for Disease Control and Prevention.* Accessed January 24. https://www.cdc.gov/tobacco/data_statistics/fact_sheets/fast_facts/index.htm.

[40] "Public Health Resources for Tobacco Control Professionals." 2019. *U.S. Food and Drug Administration.* Accessed January 24. https://www.fda.gov/TobaccoProducts/PublicHealthEducation/HealthInformation/ucm454411.htm.

[41] "Tobacco Control Act of 2009 | Public Health Law Center." 2019. *Publichealthlawcenter.Org.* Accessed January 24. https://publichealthlawcenter.org/topics/special-collections/tobacco-control-act-2009.

[42] "Products, Ingredients & Components." 2019. *FDA.gov.* Accessed January 25. https://www.fda.gov/TobaccoProducts/Labeling/ProductsIngredientsComponents/ucm20081732.htm.

[43] Benowitz, Neal L, and Jack E Henningfield. 2013. "Reducing the Nicotine Content to Make Cigarettes Less Addictive." *Tobacco Control* 22 (suppl 1): i14-i17. doi:10.1136/tobaccocontrol-2012-050860.

[44] "About Tobacco Harm Reduction – CASAA." 2019. *CASAA*. Accessed January 25. http://www.casaa.org/what-is-tobacco-harm-reduction/.

[45] "At-A-Glance." 2019. *Altria.Com.* Accessed January 25. http://www.altria.com/harm-reduction/at-a-glance/Pages/default.aspx.

In: New Research on Tobacco
Editor: Uta Dreher
ISBN: 978-1-53617-077-1

Chapter 2

TOBACCO, ITS USES AND RELEVANCE IN BASIC AND APPLIED SCIENCES: A COMPREHENSIVE OVERVIEW

Raman Manoharlal*[1,*]*, PhD, G. V. S. Saiprasad*[1]*, PhD and Ales Kovařík*[2]*, PhD

[1]Corporate R&D (Agrisciences), ITC Limited,
ITC Life Sciences and Technology Centre (LSTC),
Peenya Industrial Area, 1st Phase, Bengaluru, Karnataka, India
[2]Academy of Sciences of the Czech Republic,
Institute of Biophysics, Brno, Czech Republic

ABSTRACT

Cultivated tobacco (*Nicotiana tabacum* L.) indigenous to North and South America, is the most widely grown commercial non-food cash crop across the world. The characteristic and unique features of tobacco plant include its leaf as commercial-value, short-duration, ability to grow quickly on soils even unsuitable for other crops, relatively resistant to

* Corresponding Author's Email: ramanpdf01@gmail.com, raman.m@itc.in.

insect-pests attack, relatively easy to harvest, yields millions of seeds/plant and readily amenable to the good agricultural practices. Owing to characteristic nicotine content, tobacco leaves are commercially grown and processed into various tobacco products. Conventionally, tobacco is used in the manufacture of various 'smoke' and 'smokeless' products. Most of the scientific literature on tobacco is also devoted to industrial cigarettes manufacturing. Nevertheless in recent times, tobacco as an alternate source for various food and personal care products, paper industries, biofuel etc. has been exploited. Apart from this, tobacco plant has been also used as an excellent model for biological research in gaining fundamental knowledge in diverse areas of plant-biology. Over the past few decades, major pioneering investigations in plant-science *viz.* genetic-engineering, transgenic research, post-harvest technology, tissue-culture, nutrition and plant-growth, genetics, plant-breeding, photosynthesis, photo-periodism, biochemistry, cytology, molecular-biology, molecular-genetics, parasexual-hybridization, polyploidization, evolutionary-biology, phylogenetic, phytopathology, virology, genomics, choloroplast-genomics, epigenetics, organic-metabolism, molecular-pharming and others areas as well, owe their inception to experimentation with tobacco plants. Besides, tobacco has an incredible history to utilize as an efficient bio-factory for the valuable source of numerous phytochemicals with agricultural, pharmaceuticals and industrial applications. Realizing the enormous potential of tobacco to the mankind, this chapter is a comprehensive overview of tobacco and its application in basic and applied sciences. The purpose of this chapter is to compile and cherish the important discoveries in tobacco research and encourage researchers and scientists to continue using tobacco as a research tool because of wealth of existing scientific information about it and great potential for yet so unexplored benefits and application.

Keywords: Tobacco, *Nicotiana*, *N. tabacum*, Tobacco cultivation, Tobacco Uses, Alternative use of tobacco, Model plant, Molecular-Pharming, Basic and Applied Science

INTRODUCTION

Tobacco appears to be as old as human civilization (Goodman 1993; Borio 2001; Hanafin and Clancy 2015). The roots of tobacco cultivation dates back to many thousands of years and researchers are still trying to understand its evolutionary history and its co-evolutionary relationship with humans (Goodspeed 1954). As per ancient records, tobacco cultivation probably dates back to 8000 years when two species of the plant, *Nicotiana tabacum* L. and *N. rustica* L., were dispersed by American Indians through the Southern and Northern American continent (Mowery et al. 2015). Tobacco seeds discovered in archaeological excavations in Mexico and Peru and the remains of permanent settlements build around 3500 B.C. showed that tobacco was an important agriculture produce to the inhabitants (Luthra et al. 1992). It has been hypothesized that domestication of tobacco (genus *Nicotiana*) has possibly laid the foundation for the farming of maize and other food crops (Winter 2000). In today's world, tobacco is undeniably one of the most important non-food and high-valued cash crop cultivated globally (Johnson 1984). Based on botanical literature, tobacco is described as self to often cross-pollinated, annually-grown herbaceous plant of ~3-6 feet height with branching near the top and having large, thin and oval-shaped leaves; long fibrous taproot system consisting of primary, lateral and adventitious roots; erect, round, hairy and viscid stem and white, cream, pink or red tubular appearance flowers in large clusters (Goodspeed 1954; Breedlove and Laughlin 1993; Joshi 2018).

Tobacco-farming involves a series of agricultural practices starting from sowing in nursery, transplantation, harvesting, curing (drying/inanition), grading and bailing, followed by product-manufacturing and marketing (Figure 1 and 2). Tobacco plants are easy to grow and have a short growing-period of 90-115 days (Garner 1951; Joshi 2018). It is cultivated similar to other agricultural crops. Tobacco is propagated by seed. It is recommended that tobacco should be raised in green-houses and/ garden-sheds in nursery to obtain seedlings and subsequently about 45-60 days old healthy seedlings (ranging from 3-6 inches height) should be transplanted to the main-field (Garner 1951; Joshi 2018). The characteristic advantage of tobacco cultivation lies in its flexibility in planting time as compared to other crops. Generally, 10 g of healthy tobacco seed are sufficient to produce enough seedlings to plant one hectare (~2.47 acres) (Hartana and Vermeulen 2016). In main-field, tobacco can be grown in various soil types ranging from light (sandy), medium (loamy) and heavy (clay) soils, with pH tolerance of both acidic and basic soils and preference towards rich and well-drained moist soil under sunny condition (Joshi 2018). It cannot grow in the shade (PFAF 2014). Tobacco, being tropical in origin, but can be grown successfully under tropical, subtropical and temperate climates (Langer and Hill 1991). Today, tobacco is grown worldwide from 45° N to 40° S latitude under a wide range of climatic and edaphic conditions (Joshi 2018). Depending upon the cultivars, tobacco generally requires about 100-120 days frost-free climate with an average temperature of 20-30 °C from date of transplanting to full-maturity (Garner 1941). Tobacco is a short-day plant, thereby needing less than the critical duration of light (about 8-10 h) and a continuous dark period (about 14-16 h) in order to induce flowering (Smykal et al. 2004). Cultivated tobacco is hermaphrodite, having both male and female organs (PFAF 2014). Tobacco, typically a night-flowering plant, harbors flowers that are sweetly scented and release most of their fragrance in the evening to attract the pollinators i.e., bees and lepidoptera (moths and butterflies) (Kessler et al. 2010). Tobacco is prolific seed producer (~3000 seeds/capsule) (Erickson et al. 2013). Depending on the type, each tobacco plant produces ~14 g (~1.5-2 millions) seeds which could provide the seedlings for ~1.5 ha (3.7 acres) of field tobacco (Rao et al. 2005). Decapitation of plants at the time of blossoming i.e., 'topping' and removal of branches that subsequently develop thorough loss of apical dominance i.e., 'suckering,' are special agronomical practices followed at tobacco maturity stage (Biglar and Dehghan 2014). Tobacco is leaf-crop mainly utilized for its physiological action i.e., combustion, because of its unique 'fire-holding capacity' to glow without flame when ignited (Haley et al. 1928). Ideal conditions required for successful production of high-quality leaves are liberal and well-distributed rainfall during active vegetative growth stage, long-day length with mean temperature of 26 °C and a relatively high humidity of 70-80% during the growing season (Garner 1941; Joshi 2018). In general, tobacco plant is remarkably sensitive to the environment, wherein the commercial value of the foliage leaves (as characterized by type and quality, grade, size, shape, color, venation, elasticity, combustibility and the details of minute structure and chemical composition etc.) depends on the environment in which it is produced (Garner 1941). Apart from this, the final quality of tobacco leaves are also determined by several factors including cultivar and method of curing after harvesting (McCants and Woltz 1967). Thus, the varying conditions under which tobacco is grown resulted in localization and specialization in certain types of grades for particular tobacco products. Largely for this reason, with certain exceptions, tobacco lacks uniformity in type and quality globally, and only a relatively small portion is of commercial importance. The green leaves are excised or 'primed' as they matures [as in case of Flue-Cured Virginia (FCV) tobacco] or entire top is removed and hang in the barn for air-curing (as in case of Burley tobacco), wherein a roughly regulated regime of ventilation, temperature and humidity for the slow drying of leaves, followed by 'ageing' and 'fermentation' favours the series of physical, chemical and catabolic processes that causes the destruction of irritating ingredients and development of peculiar pleasing taste and aroma (Frankenburg 1946; Daheng et al. 1999). Notably, Cavendish and Perique tobaccos are also subjected to a second stage of curing known as *Fermenting* or *Sweating*, in a casing solution containing sugar and/or flavoring agents. Cured tobacco leaves can be stored for several years. Post-curing, leaves are sorted by farmers according to their stalk-position and quality and packed them separately into bales for delivery to the point of sale. Unlike other agricultural products, tobacco is easy and economical to transport as it is not easily perishable and has a low density ratio. Subsequently, the leaves are graded by expert leaf buyers who assess leaf quality by carefully checking the variations in color, texture and aroma (States 1989). Once the tobacco has been purchased, it is shipped to local processing units where the leaves are further processed, dried for uniformity and pressed into cases for shipment to manufacturing centers around the world, where it becomes part of the blends that will be used to manufacture different grading based tobacco products[1].

---

[1] For thorough information related to tobacco production and industry, readers are advised to consult the following literature, wherein tobacco cultivation, physiology, genetics, immediate post-harvest changes, curing, chemistry and marketing of all kinds of tobacco has been reviewed briefly: Garner 1909; Garner 1941; Frankenburg 1946; Garner 1949; Garner 1951; Steinberg and Tso 1958; Johnson 1984; Grise and Griffin 1988; Goodman 1993; Van Liemt 2001; Joshi 2018.

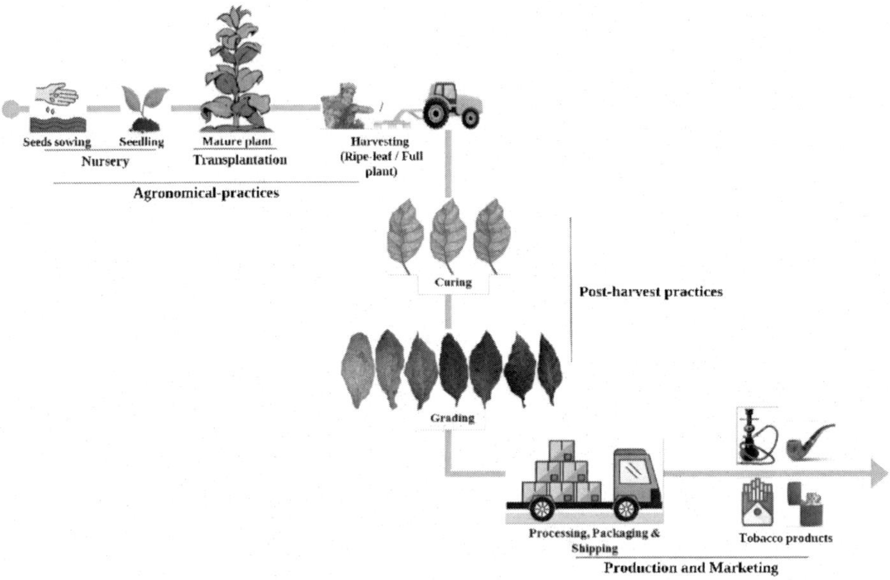

Figure 1. Tobacco-farming process. Flow-chart schematically showing the series of events involved in a typical tobacco-farming process.

TAXONOMIC AND NOMENCLATURE

Tobacco, one of the agronomically most important groups of flowering plants, belongs to extremely diverse family Solanaceae (nightshade or potato or eggplant), order Solanales and class Magnoliopsida (dicotyledons), consisting of 102 genera and 3,000-4,000 species with characteristic viscid foliage, tubular flowers and great variation in habitat, morphology and ecology (Olmstead et al. 2008). This family ranges from annual and perennial herbs to vines, lianas, epiphytes, shrubs, trees and includes some of the world's most economically important agricultural crops *viz.* medicinal, spices, weeds and ornamentals. *e.g.*, tuber-bearing potato (*Solanum tuberosum*); fruit-bearing vegetables such as tomato (*S. lycopersicum* L.), eggplant (*S. melonena* L.) and pepper (*Capsicum annum* L.); edible leaves (*S. aethiopicum* L., *S. macrocarpon* L.); ornamentals petunia (*Petunia hybrida hort.*) and angel's trumpet (*Brugmansia* sp.);

berries (*Physalis* sp.) and some deadliest plant species *viz.* belladonna (*Atropa belladonna* L.), mandrakes or Satan's apple (*Mandragora officinarum* L.), jimsonweed (*Datura stramonium* L.) and henbane (*Hyoscyamus niger* L.) (Mueller et al. 2005). There is no written record in reference to tobacco prior to 15th century. Christopher Columbus was first European person to be introduced to tobacco when he was given tobacco as a gesture of friendliness by the inhabitants of the Americas in 1492 (Borio 2001). Tobacco genus *Nicotiana* and its active principle, nicotine were named in honor of Jean Nicot de Villemain, French ambassador to Portugal who imported tobacco seeds from America to Europe in 1560 and offered it as a medicinal gift to French royal family of queen Catherine de' Medici (Borio 2001). Hence, tobacco was introduced to Europe with name *Herbe de l'ambassadeur*. The queen later renamed tobacco *Herba Regina* or *Herba Medicea*. In recognition of Nicot's role in popularizing the plant, the French botanist Jacques Dalechamps named it as *Herba Nicotiana* in the year 1586 (Borio 2001). By the end of the 16th century, tobacco use had become a custom among fashionable people in Europe. Tobacco was the first cash crop grown for money in 1612 by John Rolfe, an 'ardent smoker' and the settlers of the first American colony in Jamestown, Virginia in North America (Salmon and Salmon 2013). By 1620, tobacco was commercially grown and exported from Virginia and other American colonies to Europe (Laws 2010). Tobacco was subsequently exported to India, China and Japan (Mayne 1860; Motherby 1791). The term *Nicotiana* was used by Adam Lonitzer in 1630 to describe tobacco plants and by Carl von Linné (Linnaeus) in 1788 to designate the entire genus and thus introduced the tobacco to botany (Lonitzer and Uffenbach 1630; von Linné 1788). Commercial production of tobacco was soon extended to each and every corner of the world (Eriksen et al. 2015). Tobacco was named after Tobago, the island in the West Indies from where the major part of the tobacco used in Europe was imported (Borio 2001). Subsequently, 'Tobacco' as generic term has been used for all the products manufactured from tobacco leaves i.e., cigars, cigarettes, snuff, pipe and chewing tobacco etc.

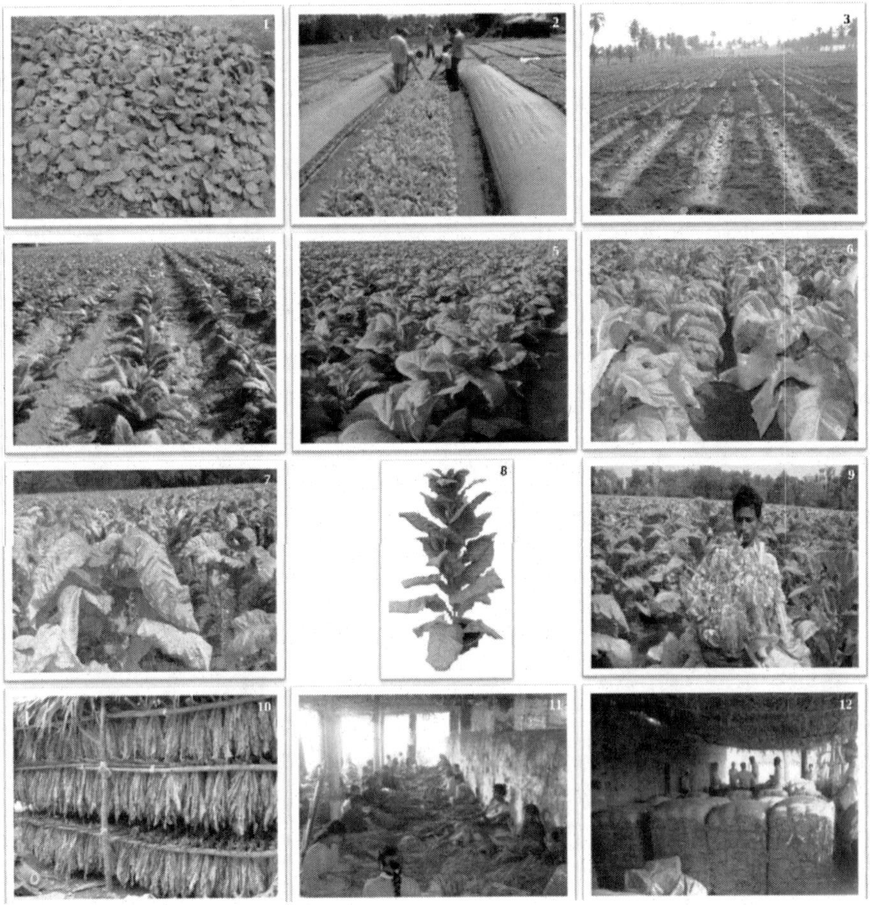

Picture courtesy: Tobacco growers, farmers and field-workers from the agronomical-fields of Rajahmundry, Andhra Pradesh (A.P.), India.

Figure 2. Depiction of various agronomical stages (from sowing to curing) in tobacco-production. 1. Tobacco seeds sowing in nursery; 2. Nursery-bed management practice; 3. Transplantation in main-field; 4. Tobacco in main-field 35 days after transplantation (DAT); 5. 55 DAT; 6. 85 DAT; 7. 125 DAT; 8. Representative picture of mature tobacco plant (125 DAT); 9. Mature leaf-harvesting based on leaf-position; 10. Leaf-curing, 11. Sorting, Grading and 12. Packaging of cured leaves in bales.

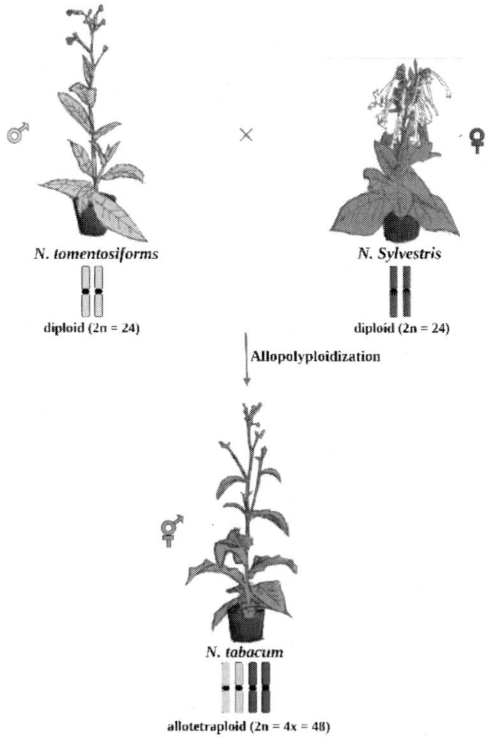

Figure 3. Genesis of *N. tabacum* L. *N. tabacum* L., a natural allotetraploid (2n = 4× = 48), has been believed to be originated by the inter-specific hybridisation of two different diploid ancestral parental species, *N. tomentosiformis* (2n = 24; paternal T genome donor) and *N. sylvestris* (2n = 24; maternal S genome donor).

A generally accepted international standard taxonomy for *Nicotiana*, referred as 'Tobacco plants,' has existed for decades which consists of 3 sub-genera, 14 sections and 66 species (Goodspeed 1954). However, most researchers now tend to classify *Nicotiana* into 13 sections and 76 species which includes 49 native to America, 25 native to Australia and 1 native to Africa (*N. africana* L.) based on size and shape of leaves and flowers (Knapp et al. 2004; Lewis and Nicholson 2007; Sierro et al. 2014). Among many important species of genera *Nicotiana*, *N. tabacum* L. is a natural allotetraploid (2n = 4× = 48), believed to be formed by inter-specific and inter-section hybridisation of two relatively divergent diploid ancestral parental species, *N. tomentosiformis* (2n = 24; section Tomentosae, paternal T genome donor) and *N. sylvestris* (2n = 24; section Sylvestres, maternal S genome donor) about 200,000 years ago (Figure 3) (Okamuro and Goldberg 1985; Arumuganathan and Earle 1991). In the Global Compendium of Weeds, *N. tabacum* L. has been listed as *Agricultural/Environmental/Noxious/Sleeper weed*, *Casual alien*, *Cultivation escape*, *Garden thug* and *Naturalised* (Randall 2012). Most of the commercial tobaccos cultivated today belong to species *N. tabacum* L. ('Common tobacco'), for which 41,600 cultivars has been listed in USDA National Plant Germplasm System, a world-famous genetic diversity warehouse for *N. tabacum* L. (USDA; https://www.ars-grin.gov/npgs/). The three most 'common tobacco' types which are traditionally grown and harvested under different agricultural practices are FCV, Burley and Oriental (Davis and Nielsen 1999). These classes differ in their genetic make-up, production, curing and use. However, all tobaccos have a common ancestral gene pool (Rufty et al. 1988; Yang et al. 2007). FCV and Burley tobaccos are the most produced and utilized classes.

A taxonomical hierarchy of cultivated tobacco (*N. tabacum* L.)

Domain: Eukaryota
- Kingdom: Plantae - Plantes, Planta, Vegetal, Plants
  - Sub-kingdom: Viridiplantae - Green plants
    - Infra-kingdom: Streptophyta - Land plants
      - Super-division: Embryophyta
        - Division: Tracheophyta - Vascular plants, Tracheophytes
          - Sub-division: Spermatophytina - Spermatophytes, Seed plants, Phanérogames
            - Class: Magnoliopsida
              - Sub-class: Dicotyledonae
                - Super-order: Asteranae
                  - Order: Solanales
                    - Family: Solanaceae - Nightshades, Solanacées
                      - Sub-family: Nicotianoideae
                        - Tribe: Nicotianeae
                          - Genus: *Nicotiana* L. - Tobacco
                            - Species: *Nicotiana tabacum* Linn. - Cultivated tobacco

Common names: Fumo, Petume, Petina, Pitura, Etum, Tabaco, Tobacco, Tabaci Folia, Tabak, Motsoko, Tootoon, Moy, May, Elder brother (Bankilal) and Angel (anjel).

Synonyms: Tabacca, Tabaci Folia, Tobacco, Tamak and Siah (Marma).

Habitat: Virginia (U.S.), China, Turkey, Greece, Holland, France, Germany and most sub-tropical countries.

TOBACCO USES[2]

The highly addictive harmala alkaloid, responsible for tobacco's narcotic and soothing qualities was isolated in 1828 and christened as 'nicotine' [synonyms: 3-(1-methyl-2-pyrrolidinyl) pyridine; (S)-(-)-nicotine; molecular formula: $C_{10}H_{14}N_2$] (Posselt and Reimann 1828). The different and conventional uses of tobacco revolve mainly around its nicotine content. Nicotine content in different *N. tabacum* varieties varies from 2-8% of the dry weight of the cured leaf, although a much larger range exists in some *Nicotiana* plants as well as species (Domino 1999). For example, a closely related *N. rustica* (called Aztek tobacco) has relatively higher content of nicotine than that of *N. tabacum*. However, except certain parts of Turkey where it is cultivated, its commercial use is low compared to cultivated tobacco. It is believed that the nicotine content is genetically controlled by two distinct loci *NICOTINE 1* and *2* (*NIC1* and *NIC2*) and corresponding mutant alleles (*nic1* and *nic2*) have been used to breed low-nicotine tobacco cultivars (Chaplin 1975; Hibi et al. 1994; Kajikawa et al. 2017b). Almost every part of the plant (except the seed) contains nicotine, but the concentration is related to different factors such as species, type of land, culture and weather conditions (Hawks Jr and Collins 1994). The concentration of nicotine increases with the age of plant. The distribution of nicotine in the mature cultivated tobacco plant is widely variable with 64% of the total nicotine exists in leaves, 18% in stem, 13% in root and 5% in flowers (Usman 2016). Tobacco leaves contain 2-8% nicotine combined as malate or citrate (Usman 2016). Owing to high nicotine content, tobacco leaves are commercially grown and processed into various tobacco products. Pure nicotine is colourless oily liquid with a boiling point of 240° F, becomes brown and crystallizes on exposure to air and dissolves in water, alcohol and oils (Brčić Karačonji 2005; Russo et al. 2011). Other related alkaloids *viz.* anabasine, anatabine and nornicotine are also present in tobacco, usually in much lower amounts (Talhout et al. 2011). Historically,

[2] Disclaimer: Tobacco should be used with great caution as it is has an addictive narcotic, nicotine. Always seek advice from the professional experts before using the tobacco for any specific purpose.

the beneficial uses of tobacco were reported to be almost endless (Wateson 1915; Monardes 1970; Hajdu and Vadmal 2010). Listed below are the various used formats of tobacco and tobacco products.

Medicinal Uses

Tobacco derived medicinal properties are the oldest form of medicine known to mankind. Once a medicinal plant and considered as *true wonder drug*, tobacco has a long recorded history of use by medical herbalists as a relaxant or analgesic (Charlton 2004). Review of literature on tobacco demonstrated that it was long used as orthodox medicine by the medical profession (Charlton 2004; Kishore 2014). Indeed, it first became known to the rest of the world when European explorers in the 15th and 16th centuries saw it being used as a medicine and as a hallucinogen by Native Americans (Borio 2001). Tobacco's medicinal as well as intoxicating properties facilitated its easy assimilation into cultural and rituals of many societies (Feinhandler et al. 1979). Although the leaves have an acrid taste, tobacco enjoyed widespread medicinal use between 16th-19th century (Charlton 2004). At least 10 *Nicotiana* species have been used in the past for ritualistic, medical or hedonistic purposes because of their intoxicating nicotine content. As is the case with many stimulants, it also have a relaxing effect on most people and seems to reduce stress (Pomerleau and Pomerleau 1991). Miraculous healing powers were attributed to tobacco plant and it was designated as *Herba Panace*, *Herba Sancta* and *Sana Sanctaindorum* (Gode 1957). It has acquired a reputation as a panacea, to the extent of being called the *Holy Herb* and *God's Remedy* (Dickson 1954). References regarding the medicinal properties of the herb tobacco were given by various workers. The ancient Indians used tobacco as a pain reliever to treat cold, skin rashes, eczema, rheumatism, toothaches, rattlesnake and insect bites (Stewart 1967). It also finds place in the synthesis of various pharmaceuticals (Tiwari et al. 2009). Tobacco waste has been used for the extraction of nicotine, the main ingredient for a wide range of drugs prescribed for conditions such as depressions, Alzheimer, Parkinson and Schizophrenia (Kuehn 2006).

Alkaloid nicotine has been also employed for the manufacture of vitamin B complex constituents, nicotinic acid and nicotinamide (Technology Information 2004). Fine ground tobacco snuff was sniffed as a remedy for cold, headache and eye problems (Stewart 1967). In Asian countries, chewing tobacco mixed with betel nuts and lime was recommended for toothache, gum diseases, aches in the throat and mental depression (Stewart 1967; Zargari 1992; Charlton 2004; Hajdu and Vadmal 2010). Decanted liquor of boiled tobacco was used internally to treat indigestion, aches in the belly and urinary obstruction (Hajdu and Vadmal 2010). Ashes of burned tobacco mixed with hog grease were applied as an ointment to ulcerated skin, warts and dermal cancer (Stewart 1967; Charlton 2004; Hajdu and Vadmal 2010). Smoking tobacco has been also claimed to improve body odour and to prevent the plague (Hajdu and Vadmal 2010). Persons of all ages and classes smoked excessively during the great epidemics. Smoking tobacco was believed to calm the nerves and relieve anxiety by purging the brain (Hajdu and Vadmal 2010). Tobacco smoke blown into the ear cured earache and when applied to the anus relieved constipation and bloody discharge (Stewart 1967; Charlton 2004; Hajdu and Vadmal 2010). Tobacco juice dropped into the ears has been reported to improve the deafness (Hajdu and Vadmal 2010). Tobacco-honey syrup was used to treat asthma, chest diseases, cough and syphilis (Stewart 1967; Charlton 2004; Hajdu and Vadmal 2010). Dried leaves, stalks and whole tobacco herb were widely used owing to their antispasmodic, discutient, diuretic, emetic, expectorant, irritant, narcotic, sedative, sialagogue, anti-inflammatory and anti-rheumatic properties (Nadkarni 1996; Iqbal et al. 2006). Tobacco pharmacological action also includes promoting evacuation of the bowel, the probable basis of its anthelmintic action (Budavari et al. 1989; Nouri et al. 2016). Several tobacco-based remedies were recognized for a wide range of gastrointestinal ailments i.e., for alleviation of painful abdominal bloating, treatment of intestinal worms, constipation and urinary stoppage (Breedlove and Laughlin 1993; Berlin and Berlin 2015). The active ingredients being readily absorbed through the skin, it has been used externally in the treatment of rheumatic swelling, skin diseases and scorpion stings (Kishore 2014). A poultice of tobacco leaves when put on skin inflammations can help soothe itching and mild pain (Stewart 1967). The nicotine in the tobacco has been reported to be responsible for drawing out the allergens and repairing the skin until its back to normal (Stewart 1967). Wet tobacco leaves has been used as analgesic and were used as a cure for painful piles. A homeopathic remedy has been made from the tobacco dried leaves (Kishore 2014). It has been also used in the treatment of nausea and travel sickness (Charlton 2004). Other than nicotine, the tobacco plants contain a range of high-value bio-chemicals such as solanesol, tobacco proteins, pectin, organic acids which can be used for the treatment of heart diseases, cancers and ulcers. Similarly, tobacco metabolites, rutin has potential applications in breast cancer therapy (Iriti et al. 2017). Despite all these aforementioned benefits, medicinal use of tobacco gradually decreased in the 1800s and was majorly replaced by the habit of smoking for pleasure. Following the scientific revelations of the mid-20th century, tobacco has been condemned as a health hazard and eventually removed from pharmacopoeias and medical practices. At present, tobacco is seldom employed internally or externally and cannot be considered a medicinal plant anymore. Nevertheless, tobacco renaissance can be expected and will certainly be fuelled by production of drugs and vaccines through ‘molecular-pharming’ and yet undiscovered medicinal properties of its secondary metabolites.

‘Smoke’ and ‘Smokeless’ Tobacco

The history of tobacco cultivation was initially concentrated on its ornamental and medicinal attributes and later only expanded for smoking purposes (Goodman 1993; Hajdu and Vadmal 2010; Kishore 2014). The consumption of tobacco among human beings has been documented since 600 A.D. (Hughes 2000), whereas it has been more than 140 years since the first mass-marketed cigarettes were produced (Wipfli and Samet 2016). In today’s world, tobacco is an industrial-crop grown mainly for ‘smoke’ and ‘smokeless’ tobacco products. Tobacco is widely used globally as a stimulant in numerous, often ritualistic manners ranging from smoking cigarettes and cigars through snorting as snuff to chewing (Hanafin and

Clancy 2015). Cured tobacco leaves are smoked, chewed or sniffed (as snuff) for their taste and flavor, but more particularly for stimulating and mildly narcotic effects of the alkaloid nicotine (Benowitz 2010). Among the various *Nicotiana* species cultivated mainly either as ornamental garden plants or as a weed, only *N. rustica* L. and *N. tabacum* L. are of economic interest. *N. rustica* L. is preferred mainly for hookah-smoking (water pipes), chewing and sniffing (Hanafin and Clancy 2015). *N. tabacum* L. is grown predominantly for 'smoke-inhalation' (*viz.* bidis, cigarettes, pipes, cigars and flavoured shisha tobacco) and 'smokeless-tobacco' (*viz.* snus, sniffed, sucked, chewed or dipping tobacco products) (Hanafin and Clancy 2015). Different cultivars or varieties of *N. tabacum* L. with different characteristics associated with smoking (*e.g.*, fast burning, slow burning, mild and strong) have become popular in different parts of the world. Based on the curing-method, 'common tobacco' has been broadly divided as flue-, fire-, air- or sun-cured (Garner 1949). In general, the dark-colored air- and fire-cured tobacco is used for pipe- and cigar-tobacco, whereas the light-colored flue- and sun-cured is used for cigarette-tobacco (Garner 1951; Davis and Nielsen 1999). More than 90% of all tobacco manufactured into cigarettes uses mainly flue-cured, broad-leaf Virginia (mild), and to some extent air-cured Burley (thin-leafed) or Maryland types, which has stronger flavor and often used for blending (Garner 1949; Jeffrey and Tso 1955). Although to a very limited extent, aromatic or oriental or Turkish tobacco having milder flavor and less nicotine produced from sun-cured small-leafed Smyrna, Samsun and Virginia types, has been also used in American Blend cigarettes (Garner 1949).

Insecticidal Uses

All parts of the plant (except the seed) contain nicotine, a powerful neurotoxin to insects that can be used as insecticide (Hawks Jr and Collins 1994). Crude tobacco extracts referred as *Ecological* or *Green pesticide*, was first used as an insecticide in 1763 as a remedy for plant lice in France (Goodman 1993). In 1828, Wilhelm Heinrich Posselt, a doctor and Karl

Ludwig Reinmann, a chemist, both from Germany, first isolated the purified nicotine from the tobacco plant and identified it's cidal-property (Posselt and Reimann 1828). Tobacco leaf extract was a popular pest control method till beginning of the 20th century (Puripattanavong et al. 2013). Tobacco dried leaves which remains effective for 6 months can also be used as insecticide (Bhattarai 1992). The juice of the leaves can be rubbed on the body as an insect repellent (Zargari 1992). Aphids, which infect plants, can also be controlled by blending soil with tobacco. Tobacco water, a traditional organic insecticide, can be used in domestic gardening (Lal and Verma 2006). Tobacco dust produced by boiling strong tobacco in water or by steeping the tobacco in water for a longer period can be used similarly. When cooled, the mixture can be applied as a spray or 'painted' on to the leaves of garden plants, where it will prove deadly to insects like aphids, peach tree borers, leaf roller, garden centipede, spiders gophers and moles (Lal and Verma 2006). Tobacco extracts has the potential to be used as organic pesticide for mangoes, vegetables and ornamentals to solve the problem of high pesticide residue (Mhazo et al. 2011). Tobacco has been also reported as organic molluscicide to control the snails and other predators as well as fertilizer to promote the growth of '*Lablab,*' natural food of fishes in fresh and brackish water (Borlongan et al. 1998).

Edible and Industrial Uses

The superior quality of tobacco protein in terms of amino acid profile and protein efficiency ratio in animal feed compared to other plant and animal proteins has been well documented (Fantozzi and Sensidoni 1983; Wildman 1983). The ability of the tobacco plant to grow in high density, yielding more than 4-fold of protein/acre than soybean, also makes it an attractive source of leaf protein in nature (Tso and Kung 1983; Tso 1990). Indeed, tobacco is the only plant from which the fraction-1-protein (F-1-p-a; single, large, homogenous protein that constitutes about 50% of soluble protein and 25% of total protein) could be extracted in pure, crystalline form (Kung 1976; Kung and Tso 1978). A highly purified F-1-p protein (99.5%

protein with no salt, fat or cholesterol) is odourless, tasteless white powder with nutritional value comparable to milk protein and casein (Sheen and Sheen 1985). F-1-p could be the best nutritional and functional food protein that can be used for manufacturing emulsifiers and high dietary supplement to cereal grains, vegetables, soft drinks and other foods (Kung et al. 1980; Wildman 1983). It can be whipped like egg whites, liquefied or gelled and can take on the flavor and texture of a variety of foods. It has been also tested as a safe protein food supplement and low calorie substitute for mayonnaise and whipped cream. In addition, malic acid (4-4.5%) and citric acid (0.5-2%) extracted from tobacco leaf can be used in foods and beverages (Sarala et al. 2013). Tobacco plant is a prolific producer of tiny seeds reaching about 1171 kg seeds/hectare, which corresponds to 432.9 kg oil/hectare (Zdremtan and Zdremtan 2006). Tobacco is indeed an oilseed crop with an oil content ranging from 30-40% of seed dry weight depending on the various agro-climatic and soil conditions (Stanisavljević et al. 2007). It has been reported that tobacco seed oil is nicotine-free, enriched in fatty acids i.e., linoleic acid (66-76%), oleic acid (17.1%), palmitic acid (7.9%) and stearic acid (3.1%) with nutritional value comparable to that of safflower oil and even better than that of groundnut and cotton seed oils (Stanisavljević et al. 2007; Sarala et al. 2013; Demirbas et al. 2016). Whenever tobacco is grown for oil-seed production, then the stalk and leaf after collection of seed could be used for the extraction of various phytochemicals and bio-actives (Grisan et al. 2016). Apart from edible purpose, tobacco seed cakes and oil also finds extensive use for animal and human alimentation as a manure and in paints, varnishes, lubricants and soap industries (Fogher 2008; Awola et al. 2010). With the invention of ever-improving mutagenesis and recombinant DNA technologies coupled with the inter-specific hybridisation followed by polyploidisation, tobacco has emerged as a promising bio-refinery crop, providing the renewable sources for the production of bio-fuels, mainly bio-ethanol (Fogher et al. 2011; Grisan et al. 2016). Indeed in the recent times, tobacco oil as a renewable source of energy in the form of 'green-energy' has been already cited as an attractive alternative to conventional tobacco products (Veljković et al. 2006; Andrianov et al. 2010; Demirbas et al. 2016; Grisan et al. 2016). Tobacco seeds contain higher quantities of biofuel oil than rapeseed and soybean (Demirbas et al. 2016). Tobacco plants have been also genetically-modified (GM) to enhance their oil content in green-tissues for the potential biofuel-production (Andrianov et al. 2010; Vanhercke et al. 2014). Generally, for producing good quality smoking/chewing leaf, tobacco plant is topped resulting in no commercial supply of seeds. However contrary to this conventional approach, an Italian research and development Sunchem Holding company has developed an elite cross-bred, non-GMO, 'Energy-Tobacco' variety called as 'Solaris' (Italian patent RM2007A000129 and international patent PCT/IB/2007/053412) which in comparison to traditional smoking tobacco, contains no nicotine in the leaves and maximizes the production of flowers/seeds with limited leaf-production (Fogher 2008). Solaris seeds possesses 33-34% of oil and the residual 67% can be used for a protein cake, thus making it highly suitable for bio-gas (electricity, biodiesel and jet fuel for aviation) and feed-industry (Fogher et al. 2011; Rossi et al. 2013). In addition, a significant quantity of capsules separated from Solaris seeds and the residual green-tissues (stems and leaves) in the field can be collected for bio-mass (paper and pulp) production. Moreover, the re-sprouting from the stump after threshing makes multiple seed harvests (up to three times a year) possible for this variety in optimal environmental and agronomical conditions.

Next-Generation Tobacco Uses

With nicotine being offending constituent and in view of apprehensions about tobacco use, the crop needs to be sustained by taking advantage of its potential for alternative uses. Moreover, the economic life-line of millions of people world-over also depends on tobacco. Thereby, to convert this threat into an opportunity in recent time researchers across the globe intensified their efforts in channelizing the tobacco into non-conventional and economically-viable alternatives (Wildman 1983; Sarala et al. 2013; Grisan et al. 2016). In this context, tobacco absolute, a kind of aromatic oil extracted from the tobacco leaves having a characteristic aroma, emerges as

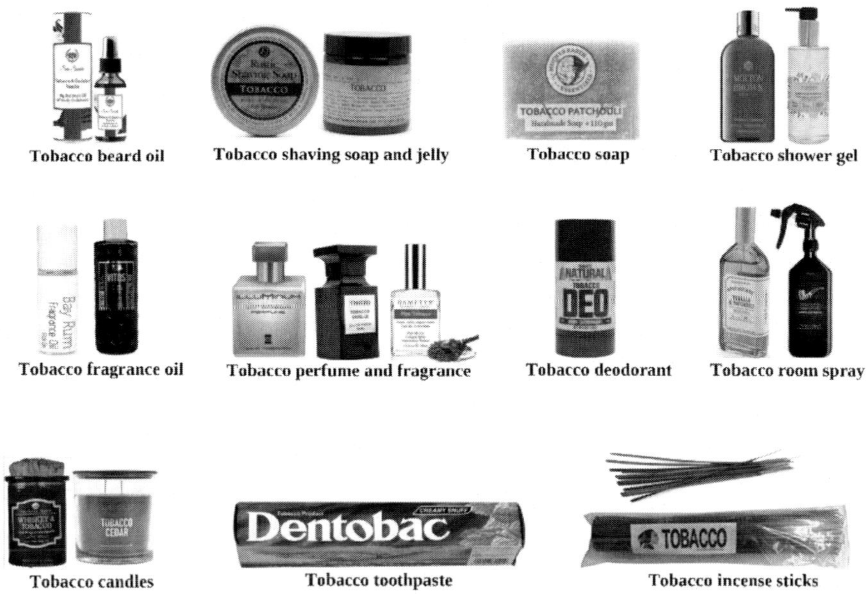

Figure 4. Next-generation tobacco products. Pictorial-representation of various tobacco based alternative-products available in global market.

a safer commercial bet. Its major component includes fuajacol, ketenes, furfural, phenols, solanesol and traces of nicotine (Gao et al. 2011; Zhang et al. 2012). Tobacco absolute without nicotine (referred as 'blond') can be used in smoking-cessation products as a component of nicotine replacement therapy (NRT) to overcome the nicotine withdrawal symptoms (*viz.* irritability, depression, restlessness, insomnia, anxiety, hunger and poor concentration) and other disorders as described in 'Diagnostic and Statistical Manual of Mental Disorders-Fourth edition' (DSM-IV) (West et al. 2006; Hartmann-Boyce et al. 2018; Yudov 2018). Instead of smoking a cigarette, smelling the tobacco absolute through each nostril helps in stopping the craving. Owing to its intense rich, warm and earthy aroma, tobacco absolute has been also employed as a base note in perfumery (Yudov 2018), adding its touch in 'dry' or 'masculine' scented perfumes, scents, soaps, shampoos, incense sticks, scented candles, room fresheners and toiletry products like toothpaste and deodorant (sclareol) etc. (Figure 4). It can also be used as biologically active component in various skin-care and cosmetic-products (*viz.* talcum powder, creams, gels and ointments etc.) for curing of acne, wrinkles, pimples, blemishes and scars (Braun 2016). It also has an 'aphrodisiac' property, which could provide effective relief to the patients suffering from the sexual problems (Braun 2016). The aqueous extract of tobacco biomass possesses significant prebiotic activity i.e., it stimulates the growth of bacteria which are beneficial to the health of human or animal gastrointestinal tracts (Akpinar et al. 2010). Two promising co-products, 'fermentable-sugars' and 'prebiotic oligosaccharides' has been recovered from tobacco (Gullón et al. 2011). Also, tobacco waste is probably the only measurable source of solanesol, an isoprenoid alcohol, an intermediary in the preparation of cardiac drugs and in the development of novel hybrid natural products such as anti-diabetic and wound-healing agents (Rowland et al. 1956; Srivastava et al. 2009; Yan et al. 2015). Rutin, a high value anti-cancer quercetin glycoside has been isolated from tobacco leaves (0.2-0.7 g/kg biomass) using a non-optimized procedure (Keinänen et al. 2001; Buyel et al. 2015). Other non-conventional tobacco products include use of ligno-cellulosic materials from tobacco-stalk as a source of cellulose and nano-cellulose in pulp-paper industry as well as reinforcement fiber in the production of fiber-cement (Shakhes et al. 2011; Wasanapiarnpong et al. 2015). Likewise, scientists from Qingdao Institute of Bioenergy and Bioprocess Technology, Chinese Academy of Sciences has developed a straightforward and inexpensive method to fabricate renewable, light-weight and water-resistant cellulose nanopaper (CNP) having potential applications in the fields of electronic devices, visual display substrates, batteries and barrier materials due to its excellent mechanical and optical properties (Wang et al. 2018). More recently, California Institute of Technology has also developed a tobacco derived sustainable and biodegradable material that possesses stiffness, strength and mechanical properties similar to and even better than the processed wood and conventional plastics (Roumeli et al. 2019). In coming years, research efforts are needed to ensure that these tobacco alternatives will become viable commercial enterprises.

SOCIO-ECONOMIC IMPACT

Tobacco use has multifactor influences. Tobacco-farming, being a highly labor-intensive and remunerative crop, provides much higher returns than other crops grown in the region. Tobacco and tobacco products also generates enormous economic benefits in terms of farm income, revenue generation and foreign exchange earnings. Indeed, tobacco is a major economic force in more than 120 countries (ResearchAndMarkets.com 2017). Among various tobacco formats, cigarettes represent one of the most popular tobacco products being consumed globally. Historically, tobacco industry grew throughout the 1700s and exploded in 1880 when a machine was first patented to mass-produce paper cigarettes (Grise and Griffin 1988). From then on, cigarettes became much easier to produce, and this saw in the dawn of the major tobacco corporations. As per latest data, 32.4 million tons (MT) of green tobacco has been used for the production of 6.48 MT of dry tobacco in six trillion cigarettes manufactured worldwide, wherein the top five producers are China (42.3%), Brazil (11.4%), India (11.1%), United States (4.6%) and Indonesia (3.4%) (Eriksen et al. 2015; FAOSTAT 2016; Zafeiridou et al. 2018). Currently, the global cigarette market with an estimate worth of around $888 billion with contribution of 10% in overall food and beverages segment ranked 4th in the global food and beverages market (ResearchAndMarkets.com 2017, 2019). With an expected compound annual growth rate (CAGR) of nearly 4% during 2019-2024, this market is further projected to reach a value of US$ 1,124 billion by 2024 (ResearchAndMarkets.com 2019). From tobacco cultivation, curing, processing, cigarette manufacturing and distribution to use and final disposal, the tobacco industry's supply chain is global and extensive (Zafeiridou et al. 2018). Tobacco industry comprises companies and personnel engaged in the growth, preparation for sale, shipment, advertisement and distribution of tobacco and tobacco-related products. Owing to this, tobacco industry is a large-scale job-creating enterprise both in agriculture and activities involved in the manufacture and marketing of tobacco products. As per Geneva-based International Labour Organization (ILO) data, over 60 million people worldwide engaged themselves in tobacco-sector, wherein 40 million were into cultivation and leaf-processing, 20 million in cottage-industries such as hand-rolling 'bidi' or 'kretek' (pronounced 'cree-teehs,' also referred as 'clove-cigarettes') cigarettes, 1.2 million in tobacco-products manufacturing and rest were employed in tobacco-related processes and industries ranging through distribution, sales and promotional activities (ILO 2003). Overall, utilization of tobacco in various innovative formats needs to be explored further to sustain the livelihood of personnel engaged in tobacco-industries as well as in controlling the tobacco use in the present form.

TOBACCO - A RESEARCH TOOL FOR BASIC AND APPLIED SCIENCES

Basic Sciences

Being a lucrative crop, tobacco has been the research subject for commercial interest. Conventional tobacco research has been aimed at the development of improved and high yielding varieties, improved input use efficiency, post-harvest management practices and plant protection measures etc., which has made a significant impact on tobacco production, marketing and export earnings. However, on contrary to general public opinion, rather than just being a cigarette-filler, tobacco has played a significant role in modern biological research and has been most abundant source of scientific information (Tso 2006). For instance, the knowledge gained from special post-harvesting processes in tobacco *viz.* curing, aging and fermentation has been widely appreciated in enzymology, microbiology, catalytic chemistry and in tea- and wine-industries. It is now grown in green-houses and growth-chambers of research institutions, universities and biotechnology companies all over the world. Tobacco is well placed to take advantage of molecular methods for genetic-improvement (Tso 2006). Center for Tobacco Reference Products (CTRP; https://ctrp.uky.edu/) developed by Kentucky Tobacco Research and Development Center

(KTRDC), University of Kentucky, U.S., offered certified reference tobacco products as standards for non-clinical investigations (intended for research purposes only and are not for human consumption) to tobacco manufacturers, contract and government laboratories and academic institutions since 1968. U.S. FDA also supports research programs and projects that include, but are not limited to, the scientific fields of epidemiology, behavior, biology, medicine, economics, chemistry, engineering, toxicology, pharmacology, addiction, public health, communications, marketing and statistics in order to better understand the tobacco use and associated risks. Indeed, most public institutions have appropriately moved beyond the days of tobacco research as a smoke-product. Owing to readily available resources to facilitate the research in tobacco including transformation and regeneration systems, reduced complexity, cell culture lines and extensive mutant and breeding collections (Geelen and Inzé 2001), significant progress has been made in pioneering research areas, especially in the fields of tissue-culture, genetics, plant-breeding, genomics, epigenetics, biotic- and abiotic-stress physiology, chemistry, organic metabolism, evolutionary-biology, biotechnology and molecular-biology as well as other research areas (Figure 5). Listed below are the most prominent areas of basic sciences, wherein tobacco has contributed immensely.

Agricultural Biotechnology

Although *Arabidopsis thaliana* is a major model-plant in scientific community (Koornneef and Meinke 2010), it does not necessarily reflect the most representative species to address all plant phenomena. Indeed, tobacco could still be the sidekick to *A. thaliana* in plant-biology research and shines ever more brightly with realized and yet-to-be-exploited potential. The number of publications on tobacco as model system over the last decade has exceeded enormously. As of 01st October, 2019, citation count showed 3837 research articles in the NCBI PubMed database when utilising '*Nicotiana* as model system' as a search term. During the last five decades, tobacco has been widely recognized as an excellent research tool, similar to that of *Escherichia coli* and 'HeLa cells' in biological science (Nagata et al. 1992;

Ganapathi 2004; Sussex 2008). It was when using tobacco, Murashige and Skoog in 1962, revised the culture media for the propagation of plants and this nutrient formulation was later used for the *in vitro* culture of other crops (Murashige and Skoog 1962) which is the most frequently used medium till now.

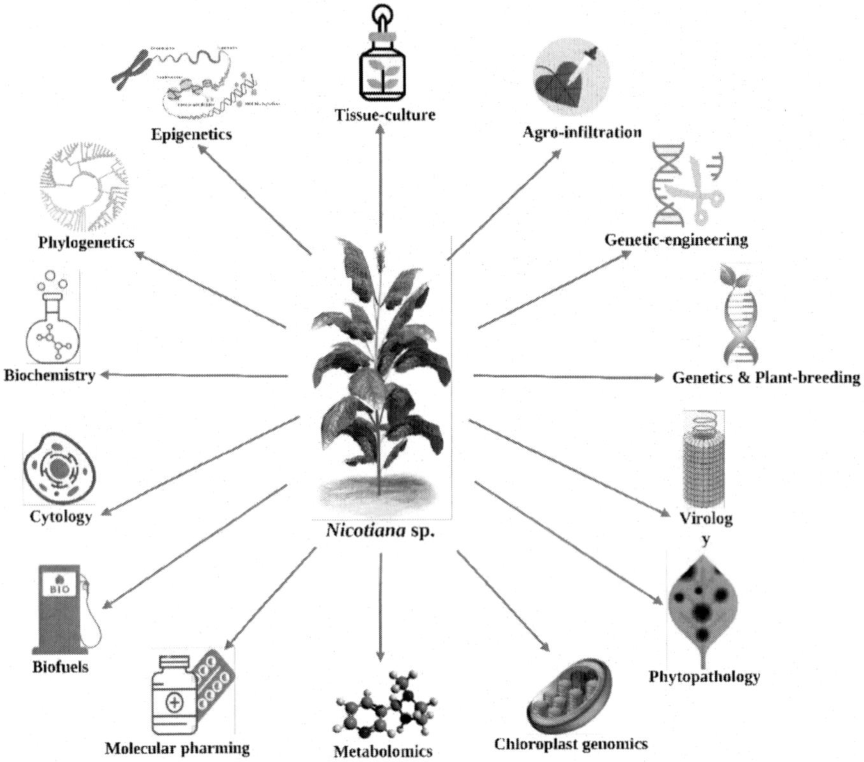

Figure 5. Tobacco, a convenient experimental system. *Nicotiana* sp. as an experimental system has been exploited in various research topics pertaining to basic and applied sciences.

Tobacco has also played a pioneering role in callus culture research and the elucidation of the mechanism by which kinetin works, laying the groundwork for modern agricultural biotechnology (Skoog and Miller 1957; Budzianowska 2009). Isolation, culture and regeneration of protoplast into a complete plant and somatic hybridisation were studied successfully in tobacco (Nagata and Takebe 1971). Being the first plant to demonstrate amenability to tissue-culture, genetic-engineering, totipotency, regeneration from protoplast, somatic-hybrid and chimera formation, *N. tabacum* L. had become the most celebrated model system for tissue-culture and genetic-engineering studies over the past several decades and continues to remain as *'Cinderella of Plant Biotechnology'* (Vasil and Hildebrandt 1965; Nagata and Takebe 1971; Nitsch and Ohyama 1971; Ogura 1976; Hoekema et al. 1983; Gadani et al. 1995). Almost all historical tissue-culture achievements *viz.* growth medium formulations, studies on growth, development, differentiation, regeneration, senescence, organogenesis, embryogenesis, growth regulators, protoplast fusion, somatic hybridization, somaclonal variations, anther and pollen culture, induction of haploids, microspore-derived embryos, mutant cell lines selection, genetic and epigenetic stability of the genome in tissue culture conditions, secondary metabolism, biotic- and abiotic-stresses has been accomplished using tobacco as model system (Pouteau et al. 1991; Hirochika 1993; Ganapathi 2004; Koukalova et al. 2005; Sussex 2008; Budzianowska 2009). Tobacco BY-2 cell line, derived from *N. tabacum* L. cultivar 'Bright Yellow-2' and NT-1 (*N. tabacum*-1) cells, are the most popular and widely used in plant research (Nagata et al. 1992; Ganapathi 2004; Budzianowska 2009). Hundreds of scientific papers have been published using this line as a model to study various aspects of plant cell physiology. These cell lines are relatively homogenous, allowing to investigate the studies of cell phenotypes and cellular responses to environmental stresses under the control conditions (Koukalova et al. 1997; Kovarik et al. 1997; Kuthanova et al. 2008; Kutik et al. 2014; Takahashi et al. 2015). They have appealing features including being fast-growing, robust, enabling synchronization of cell divisions and cell-cycle analyses (Geelen and Inzé 2001; Harashima et al. 2007; Kuthanova et al. 2008). Being easily transformable either by particle bombardment (Klein et al. 1988) or by co-cultivation with *Agrobacterium tumefaciens* (An 1985), transgenic derivatives of BY-2 and NT-1 cell lines have had high impact in analyses of protein function by ectopic-expression, gene knock-outs or translational gene fusions (Nocarova and Fischer 2009; Nair et al. 2014).

Transgenic Studies

A simple genetic-transformation method to tobacco based on leaf disc method has become standard for producing transgenic plants (Burow et al. 1990). In 1982, tobacco harbouring an antibiotic-resistant marker became the first GM plant, which laid the foundation for all GM crops (Bevan et al. 1983). Because of its importance as a research tool, herbicide resistance transgenic tobacco was the first GM crop to be tested in field trials, in the United States and France in 1986 (James 2001). In 1987, Plant Genetic Systems (Ghent, Belgium) became the first company to develop GM tobacco plants by incorporating insect resistant genes from *Bacillus thuringiensis* (Bt). In 1988, China became the first country in the world to begin growing virus-resistant GM tobacco commercially and in 1993 approved its commercial planting (Tao and Shudong 2003). In 1994, the European Union (EU) approved the herbicide bromoxynil resistant GM tobacco, thus making it as the first commercial GM crop marketed in Europe (James 2001). Subsequently, many varieties of transgenic tobacco harboring agronomic traits such as resistance to pathogens and insect-pests [viruses, particularly to the tobacco mosaic virus (TMV), fungi, bacteria and nematodes], drought, cold, herbicides and for bioremediation etc., have been intensively tested in field trials. *N. tabacum* L. has been used extensively in plant transgenic research involving disease susceptibility, response to serious pathogens (*e.g.*, Bt genes against tobacco budworm), pyridine alkaloid (like nicotine) biosynthesis, cell cycle, oxidative stress and pollen tube development etc. in order to understand the fundamental biological processes (Miki et al. 1999; Jube and Borthakur 2007).

Genetics and Breeding

Tobacco, being representative of higher plants, is also ideal for genetics and breeding studies, because of availability of many *Nicotiana* species, easy self- and cross-pollination, high success rate of interspecific-crosses, abundance and longevity of its seeds, large range of variability for most plant characters and extensive information accumulated from biometrical genetic studies (Garner 1951; Steinberg and Tso 1958; Davis and Nielsen 1999; Peedin 2002; Schaeffer et al. 2012; PFAF 2014). Thorough and extensive research in tobacco has generated a huge amount of Tobacco Genetics and Breeding database (TGB, http://biodb.sdau.edu.cn/tgb/) (Cao et al. 2013). In addition, there are many distinctive chemical, physical and botanical characteristics of tobacco that provide numerous molecular markers for scientific studies (Liu and Zhang 2008; Tong et al. 2012; 2016).

Genomics - Genome Structure and Sequence Resources

During the last few years, massive biological data have emerged from in-depth genomics studies of tobacco. In 1986, tobacco became the first plant for which complete sequence of chloroplast (cp) genome (155,943 bp) was reported (Shinozaki et al. 1986). Since then, tobacco also became the most preferred model for understanding the evolutionary relationship among photosynthetic organisms and cp (plastid)-engineering or chloroplast transformation technology (CTT) for agricultural biotechnology applications (Daniell et al. 2002; 2005). CTT brings advantages such as control of the site of gene insertion, high rates of transgene expression and protein accumulation, lack of transmission of the transgene *via* pollen due to the fact that plastid genes are maternally inherited and an absence of epigenetic effects (Daniell et al. 2004). Improving agricultural traits such as herbicide and pathogen resistance, resistance to drought and salt tolerance, phytoremediation and molecular-pharming are all promising and potential applications of CTT (Daniell et al. 2002; 2005; Řepková 2010; Adem et al. 2017). The knowledge obtained from tobacco chloroplast genome can be easily applied to over 800 complete cp genome sequences that have been made publicly available in the National Center for Biotechnology Information (NCBI) organelle genome database (http://www.ncbi.nlm.nih.gov/*genome*) that includes 300 crops (such as maize, tomato, rice, barley, carrot, cotton, papaya, pea, pine, potato, sunflower and sugar beets etc. to name a few) and tree genomes (Daniell et al. 2016), thus making tobacco as important research material for cp-genomics studies. *N. tabacum* L. genome (estimated size 4.5 GB), because of its complexity and importance, was also the focus target for SOL-100 sequencing project [Solanaceae Genomics Network (SGN); https://solgenomics.net], which aimed to decipher the genomes of most important Solanaceae species (Fernandez-

Pozo et al. 2014). Numerous coding-genes and repeated sequences of *N. tabacum* L. have been deciphered in details and a gene space library has been constructed (Rushton et al. 2008), which represented a significant step towards plant-genomics research (Sierro et al. 2013; Sierro et al. 2014). In recent times, efforts from Tobacco Genome Initiative (TGI) provided the draft genome sequences for *N. tabacum* L. as well as its ancestral parents (http://www.tobaccogenome.org/), thus further making it a convenient model-system for genetic-manipulation. As with most other plant species (Heslop-Harrison and Schwarzacher 2011), a large fraction of *Nicotiana* genome is comprised of various types of retroelements. Genome sampling using next generation sequencing (NGS) revealed that the major component of *N. tabacum* genome and its diploid relatives comprises long terminal repeat (LTR)-retrotransposons (Renny-Byfield et al. 2011), with 17.1-22.5% and 2.2-3.4% of genome being Ty3/gypsy and Ty1/copia elements, respectively. DNA transposons comprise around 1.7% of the genome of these species. In addition, there are several unrelated satellite repeat families that have been characterized and used as convenient chromosome markers. These repeats include: (1) The HRS60 family, which is the best characterised tandem repeat family in *Nicotiana*, and includes an interstitial repeat in *N. tomentosiformis* and *N. tabacum* (called GRS) and predominantly subtelomeric repeats in *N. sylvestris* and *N. tabacum* (called HRS60, NSYL2) (Koukalova et al. 2010; Koukalova et al. 1989; Gazdova et al. 1995) (2) NTS9 in *N. sylvestris* and *N. tabacum* (Jakowitsch et al. 1998); (3) NTRS and NiCL3 tandem repeats in *N. tomentosiformis* and *N. tabacum* (Matyasek et al. 1997; Renny-Byfield et al. 2012); (4) A family of (peri)centromeric tandem satellites; HT3E06, HT1H04 and HT3G02 (Shibata et al. 2013). There are also a number of satellite repeat families of known origin, these are: (5) A1/A2 satellite repeats derived from the intergenic spacer (IGS) of 18-5.8-26S nuclear ribosomal (rDNA), which have transposed and amplified to multiple locations across the genome (Lim et al. 2004b); (6) Tandem repeats of geminivirus related DNA (GRD), occurring in two distinct families in some accessions of *N. tomentosiformis* and inherited to *N. tabacum* (Murad et al. 2002). These sequences are also the first endogenous viruses discovered in plants (Bejarano et al. 1996) and

(8) Sequences of retroviral (Nagaki et al. 2011) and pararetroviral origin (Matzke et al. 2004).

Epigenetics

Apart from genomics, tobacco has also garnered the attention of several investigations pertaining to plant-epigenetics studies over the last three decades (Grant-Downton and Dickinson 2005; Meyer 2005). *N. tabacum* L., being a natural and classic allotetraploid crop, displays wide environmental adaptability as a result of many years of extensive artificial cross-breeding, mainly through epigenetic regulation, represents an important model of higher-plant for epigenetic studies (Comai 2000; Murad et al. 2002; Liu and Wendel 2003; Sutherland and Costa 2003; Lim et al. 2004a). Epigenetic mechanisms involved in chromatin dynamics, DNA methylation and histone modification patterns etc., leading to an appreciation of how new phenotypes could be generated quickly in response to environmental modifications mainly *via* transcriptional and post-transcriptional gene-silencing, has been dissected using tobacco as a model system (Schmitt et al. 1997; Boyko and Kovalchuk 2011; Křížová et al. 2013; Manoharlal et al. 2018a; 2018b; Wang et al. 2018; Manoharlal et al. 2019). Several epigenetic genes including 5-methylcytosine DNA methyltransferases (Nakano et al. 2000; Wada et al. 2003; Kim et al. 2007; Fulneček et al. 2009; Lin et al. 2015) has been isolated and functionally characterised (Nakano et al. 2000; Kim et al. 2007; Lin et al. 2015) using tobacco as a case-study. With the advent of robust methods and ever improving next-generation tools and technologies, the popularity of this much-cherished model plant is anticipated to see a continuous and further rise in plant-genomics and -epigenetics research.

Evolutionary Studies

Nicotiana species also serves as an excellent model for investigating the plant polyploidy. Polyploidy i.e., the merging of more or less divergent genomes associated with whole genome duplication, is an important factor in eukaryote evolution (Otto and Whitton 2000; Lynch and Walsh 2007). The discovery of tobacco polyploid genome goes back to the mid of the last century where cytogeneticists identified a double amount ($2n = 4\times = 48$) of chromosomes in its karyotype and subsequent back-crossing experiments revealed its hybridogenic origin (Goodspeed 1954; Gerstel 1963). Kenton *et. al.* (1993) was the first to use genomic *in situ* hybridization (GISH) to study the genome structure of *N. tabacum* (Kenton et al. 1993). The fluorescent probes derived from the total genomic DNA of each *N. sylvestris* and *N. tomentosiformis* preferentially hybridized to a subset of 24 chromosomes of *N. tabacum*, corresponding to the chromosomes of the S- and T-genomes respectively. Subsequent molecular markers analysis based on endogenous geminiviruses (Murad et al. 2002), amplified fragment length polymorphism (AFLP) patterns (Ren and Timko 2001) and retroelements (Petit et al. 2007) have further narrowed the origin of the tobacco paternal genome donor to a particular lineage of *N. tomentosiformis*. Important advancements and numerous evolutionary changes such as elimination of tandem repeats (Skalicka et al. 2005; Renny-Byfield et al. 2011), inter-genomic translocations (Kenton et al. 1993; Moscone et al. 1996; Lim et al. 2004a), gene conversion of rDNA (Volkov et al. 1999), activation of a subset of transposable elements (Petit et al. 2010) have been reported in tobacco genome. These changes have been mostly bound to the paternal T-genome, while the maternal S-genome seems to be more stable lending some support for the nucleo-cytoplasmatic hypothesis (Gill and Friebe 2013). Recently, whole genomic studies began to reveal allopolyploidy related changes not only in repeated (mostly non-coding) fraction of tobacco genome, but also in protein-coding genes (Kajikawa et al. 2017a; 2017b; Siminszky et al. 2007). Interestingly, one of the mutations apparently stimulated accumulation of nicotine in tobacco but not in its progenitors (Chakrabarti et al. 2007). All these findings in polyploidy research have been elucidated using tobacco as case-studies, which pave the path in recognizing the major implications in evolution of plants, especially by promoting genetic diversity, adaptive radiation and speciation (Lim et al. 2004a; 2004b; Dadejová et al. 2007; Bombarely et al. 2012; Tayalé and Parisod 2013). Being an allotetraploid, tobacco also serves as convenient 'aneuploidy' model system to follow the fate of genes present on a homeologous chromosome(s) through growth and sexual reproduction (Papp et al. 1996).

Virology

The economic impact of tobacco mosaic disease led to the isolation, purification and structural characterization of first simplest virus (i.e., TMV), which laid the foundation and rapid advancement in the field of virology (Bawden et al. 1936; Franklin et al. 1958; Stanley 1935). Owing to hyper-susceptibility to a wide variety of plant viruses and other plant-pathogenic agents (bacteria, oomycetes, fungi etc.) and also the rapidity with which visible phenotypes appears, *N. benthamiana* L., Benth (or Benthi) as it is colloquially known, a dwarf and closely related species to *N. tabacum* L., is one of the most commonly used model plant by the virology community for host-pathogen interaction studies, particularly in the context of innate-immunity and defense-signaling (Goodin et al. 2008; Bally et al. 2018). Moreover, being amenable to genetic-transformation with good regeneration efficiency and facile methods for virus-induced gene silencing (VIGS), *N. benthamiana* L. has been also extensively exploited in the development of viral vectors that can express foreign-genes and the establishment of VIGS, which enabled the knocking down of plant endogenous genes (Goodin et al. 2008). The fact that *A. thaliana* not ideal for the systemic processes and fast transient methods (*viz.* agro-infiltration or VIGS) that enabled transient protein expression, *N. benthamiana* L. based agro-infiltration also became the method of choice in cell biology, biochemistry and other *in planta* studies, wherein particular studies requires the protein localization, protein-protein interactions or plant-based systems for protein expression and purification (Daròs and Flores 2004; Wroblewski et al. 2005; Goodin et al. 2008).

Applied Sciences

Instead of drying the tobacco leaves to make cigarettes, tobacco can be used for other purposes that are beneficial for health. Since the first human protein (serum albumin) was expressed in tobacco cells in 1990 (Sijmons et al. 1990), a wide array of bio-actives has been successfully produced in tobacco plant during past 3 decades. In recent times, research with tobacco plants has already imparted an important contribution in applied sciences, far beyond the frontiers of agricultural-science. Owing to its unique advantages over other plant species i.e., relatively short generation-time (4 months from seed to next-generation seed), ease of cultivation, field-level scalability (scalable to thousands of acres), bulk leaf-production, ability to express proteins in bulk (>40% of its dry weight) at commercial-levels (~2 tons protein/acre/yr) without the need of flowering, high metabolic versatility (>4,000 metabolites), negligible risks of outcrossing with native wild relatives, non-food status with minimum possibility of contamination with industrial-designated products and amenability to genetic-transformation, tobacco is currently one of the most appropriate 'chassis' to be used as 'molecular-pharming'/'green-bioreactor' platform (Steinberg and Tso 1958; Tso 1990; Rymerson et al. 2002; Ganapathi 2004; Horn et al. 2004). Researchers, biotechnology companies and bioengineering entrepreneurs have found cutting-edge new plant-breeding techniques to turn tobacco leaves into efficient plant factories for medical, pharmaceutical and cosmetic products (Spiegel et al. 2018). Numerous initiatives has been successfully established for the production of wide range of 'biopharmaceuticals' *viz.* recombinant-proteins; industrial proteins and enzymes (*e.g.,* avidin, β-casein, liquid crystal polymers, xylanase xyloglucanases, anthranilate synthase, endo- and exo-cellulases, β-glucosidases, pectate lyases, cutinases, acetylcholine esterase and horseradish peroxidase *etc.*); pharmaceutical-proteins (*e.g.,* human somatotropin, serum albumin, interferon and monoclonal antibodies *etc.*); vaccines against bacterial- (cholera, tetanus, anthrax, small pox and Lyme disease) and viral-pathogens (canine parvovirus and rotavirus); cytokines [*e.g.,* human interferon γ or interleukin-18 (INF-γ or IL-18)]; steroids; alkaloids; phenolics and vitamins *etc.* (Gadani et al. 1995; Cramer et al. 1996; Rymerson et al. 2002; Ma et al. 2003; Ganapathi 2004; Paul et al. 2011; Kaldis et al. 2013; Ma et al. 2015). In recent times, number of companies have been established globally to exploit the inherent potential of tobacco for various purposes. For instance, Planet Biotechnology Inc., California, U.S. (https://www.planetbiotechnology.com) has created the first clinically advanced anti-caries monoclonal plantibody from tobacco,

CaroRx®, against *Streptococcus mutans* (Larrick et al. 1998). Dow AgroSciences LLC, Indianapolis, U.S. (www.dowagro.com) in 2006 received the world's first plant-based regulatory approval for the production of tobacco cell-based (Concert™ Plant-Cell-Produced System) vaccine against Newcastle disease virus in poultry from USDA Center for Veterinary Biologics (Fox 2006). Mapp Biopharmaceutical Inc., San Diego, U.S. (https://mappbio.com) has developed a drug, 'Zmapp' to fight the outbreak of Ebola using tobacco antibody production (Langreth et al. 2014). iBio CMO, LLC, Bryan, TX, U.S. (https://www.ibioinc.com), formerly Caliber Biotherapeutics LLC, utilizes tobacco plant-based expression system for manufacturing the recombinant proteins targeting non-Hodgkin's lymphoma, multiple myeloma and breast cancers (Holtz et al. 2015). Medicago Inc. (https://www.medicago.com), a Québec, Canada based biopharmaceutical company (subsidiary of Mitsubishi Tanabe Pharma Corporation, Japan) is developing a vaccine and therapeutic proteins for influenza called 'Proficia.' Another relevant example is the production of aprotinin in tobacco by Kentucky BioProcessing (KBP) Inc., Owensboro, U.S. (https://www.kentuckybioprocessing.com). Other leading and notable organizations involved in the production of biopharmaceuticals based on transient expression in tobacco includes Icon Genetics, Halle, Germany (https://www.icongenetics.com) and Fraunhofer Center for Molecular Biotechnology, Newark, DE, U.S. (https://www.fraunhofer.org). In this context, it is also worth mentioning here that Pharma-planta (www.plantpharma.org), a consortium of 39 academic principal investigators and industrial partners in Europe and Africa funded by the European Commission, has developed an anti-HIV antibody using tobacco as host-system (Fox 2011). In recent times, a 7.2 million Euros Horizon 2020 project, NEWCOTIANA, coordinated by scientists at Institute for Plant Molecular and Cellular Biology (IBMCP) from the Spanish Research Council (CSIC) with participation of 19 industrial and academic partners form 8 European countries and Australia has been also initiated, which aims to develop new varieties in *N. tabacum* L. and *N. benthamiana* L. to produce compounds such as antibodies, vaccines and drugs in a sustainable and commercial manner (https://newcotiana.org/). Likewise, Kentucky Tobacco

Research and Development Center (KTRDC; https://ktrdc.ca.uky.edu), University of Kentucky, U.S. also emphasizing on applications-oriented research to support the tobacco and other *Nicotiana* species as a production system for the plant-based applied products (including pharmaceuticals and industrial materials) and for discovering of novel and commercially-viable plant-based natural products.

Having said this and realising the enormous benefits of tobacco, development of economically viable and value-added tobacco products with a commitment towards better utilization of tobacco in current format requires innovative scientific interventions. To achieve this target, there is a need to constantly explore the tobacco crop through re-orientation of research efforts, policy initiatives and forging the effective collaboration with industries.

CONCLUSION

Scientifically, tobacco was the 19th century 'model' plant for understanding the plant-hybridisation, whilst during the 20th century it has been used to evaluate the fundamental plant-biology phenomenon. Contrary to general public opinion, tobacco has many valuable uses other than smoking. Tobacco was and till today, is the most abundant source of scientific information for basic sciences and a valuable commodity for applied sciences. Knowing its great potential in future, we anticipate that the use of tobacco is only at its beginning. Our present chapter is an attempt to expand and put forth a persuasive case for researchers and scientists to take up the challenge to unlock the yet hidden and unexplored plant-biology phenomenon(s) that could be derived from tobacco. We anticipate that comprehensive compilation of these studies will further consolidate the tobacco stature in plant kingdom as a versatile 'model' of higher-plants for future plant-biology studies.

Conflict of Interest Statement

All authors have read and approved the final manuscript. The authors declare that there are no conflict of interest. The content of this manuscript does not necessarily reflect the views or policies of ITC Limited, ITC Life Sciences and Technology Centre (ITC-LSTC).

Acknowledgments

We would like to acknowledge Former (Dr. C. C. Lakshmanan) and Current (Dr. Krishnan Venkateswaran) Head, Corporate R&D, ITC-LSTC) for their consistent support and encouragement. A very special thanks to Ashima Banga (Guru Nanak Dev University, Punjab, India) for her assistance in critically editing the manuscript and helpful comments. Our appreciation is also extended to tobacco growers, farmers and field-workers at Northern Light Soil (NLS) region, Rajahmundry, Andhra Pradesh (A. P.), India for providing their support, guidance during field-visit and briefings about the trade and tricks of tobacco-farming, gradings and marketing. We apologize to the many tobacco researchers whose specific and significant research work could not be mentioned in this chapter because of length constraints.

References

Adem, M., Beyene, D. and Feyissa, T. (2017). Recent achievements obtained by chloroplast transformation. *Plant Methods,* 13(1): 30.

Akpinar, O., Erdogan, K., Bakir, U. and Yilmaz, L. (2010). Comparison of acid and enzymatic hydrolysis of tobacco stalk xylan for preparation of xylooligosaccharides. *LWT-Food Science and Technology,* 43(1): 119-125.

An, G. (1985). High efficiency transformation of cultured tobacco cells. *Plant Physiology,* 79(2): 568-570.

Andrianov, V., Borisjuk, N., Pogrebnyak, N., Brinker, A., Dixon, J., Spitsin, S., et al. (2010). Tobacco as a production platform for biofuel: overexpression of *Arabidopsis DGAT* and *LEC2* genes increases accumulation and shifts the composition of lipids in green biomass. *Plant Biotechnology Journal,* 8(3): 277-287.

Arumuganathan, K. and Earle, E. (1991). Nuclear DNA content of some important plant species. *Plant Molecular Biology Reporter,* 9(3): 208-218.

Awola, V., Ogunniyi, D. and Odetoye, T. (2010). Refining, modification and characterization of tobacco seed oil for improved potentials for industrial use. *Nigerian Journal of Pure and Applied Sciences,* 23: 2168-2174.

Bally, J., Jung, H., Mortimer, C., Naim, F., Philips, J. G., Hellens, R., et al. (2018). The rise and rise of *Nicotiana benthamiana*: A plant for all reasons. *Annual Review of Phytopathology,* 56(1): 405-426.

Bawden, F., Pirie, N., Bernal, J. and Fankuchen, I. (1936). Liquid crystalline substances from virus-infected plants. *Nature,* 138(3503): 1051.

Bejarano, E. R., Khashoggi, A., Witty, M. and Lichtenstein, C. (1996). Integration of multiple repeats of geminiviral DNA into the nuclear genome of tobacco during evolution. *Proceedings of the National Academy of Sciences of the United States of America,* 93(2): 759-764.

Benowitz, N. L. (2010). Nicotine addiction. *New England Journal of Medicine,* 362(24): 2295-2303.

Berlin, E. A. and Berlin, B. (2015). *Medical Ethnobiology of the Highland Maya of Chiapas, Mexico: The Gastrointestinal Diseases*: Princeton University Press.

Bevan, M. W., Flavell, R. B. and Chilton, M. D. (1983). A chimaeric antibiotic resistance gene as a selectable marker for plant cell transformation. *Nature,* 304(5922): 184.

Bhattarai, N. (1992). Medical ethnobotany in the Karnali zone, Nepal. *Economic Botany,* 46(3): 257-261.

Biglar, P. S. S. and Dehghan, Z. H. (2014). Effects of topping and suckericide on leaf quality of tobacco (*Nicotiana tabacum*). *International journal of Advanced Biological and Biomedical Research,* 2(3): 723-731.

Borio, G. (2001). *The Tobacco Timeline.* http://www.tobacco.org/History/Tobacco_History.html

Borlongan, I. G., Coloso, R. M., Mosura, E. F., Sagisi, F. D. and Mosura, A. T. (1998). Molluscicidal activity of tobacco dust against brackishwater pond snails (*Cerithidea cingulata* Gmelin). *Crop protection,* 17(5): 401-404.

Boyko, A. and Kovalchuk, I. (2011). *Genetic and epigenetic effects of plant-pathogen iteractions: An Evolutionary Perspective.* (Vol. 4, pp. 1014-1023).

Braun, D. (2016). *Tobacco absolute (Nicotiana Tabacum)-Essential oil profile, benefits, properties.* https://www.natural-holistic-health.com/tobacco-absolute-nicotiana-tabacum-essential-oil-profile-benefits-properties/

Brčić Karačonji, I. (2005). Facts about nicotine toxicity. *Arhiv za higijenu rada i toksikologiju,* 56(4): 363-371.

Breedlove, D. E. and Laughlin, R. M. (1993). Flowering of Man: A Tzotzil Botany of Zinacantán, Volume II. *Smithsonian Contributions to Anthropology.*

Budavari, S., O'Neil, M. J., Smith, A. and Heckelman, P. E. (1989). *The merck index* (Vol. 11): Merck Rahway, NJ: Merck.

Budzianowska, A. (2009). In vitro cultures of tobacco and their impact on development of plant biotechnology. *Przeglad Lekarski,* 66(10): 890-893.

Burow, M. D., Chlan, C. A., Sen, P., Lisca, A. and Murai, N. (1990). High-frequency generation of transgenic tobacco plants after modified leaf disk cocultivation with *Agrobacterium tumefaciens. Plant Molecular Biology Reporter,* 8(2): 124-139.

Buyel, J., Buyel, J., Haase, C. and Fischer, R. (2015). The impact of Pseudomonas syringae type III effectors on transient protein expression in tobacco. *Plant Biology,* 17(2): 484-492.

Cao, H., Wang, Y., Xie, Z., Huang, L., Xu, H., Zhang, L., et al. (2013). TGB: the tobacco genetics and breeding database. *Molecular Breeding,* 31(3): 655-663.

Chakrabarti, M., Meekins, K. M., Gavilano, L. B. and Siminszky, B. (2007). Inactivation of the cytochrome P450 gene *CYP82E2* by degenerative mutations was a key event in the evolution of the alkaloid profile of modern tobacco. *New Phytologist,* 175(3): 565-574.

Chaplin, J. F. (1975). Registration of LAFC53 tobacco germplasm. *Crop Science,* 15: 282.

Charlton, A. (2004). Medicinal uses of tobacco in history. *Journal of the Royal Society of Medicine,* 97(6): 292-296.

Comai, L. (2000). Genetic and epigenetic interactions in allopolyploid plants. In *Plant Gene Silencing* (pp. 267-279): Springer Dordrecht.

Cramer, C. L., Weissenborn, D. L., Oishi, K. K., Grabau, E. A., Bennett, S., Ponce, E., et al. (1996). Bioproduction of human enzymes in transgenic tobacco a. *Annals of the New York Academy of Sciences,* 792(1): 62-71.

Daheng, Z., Jinfeng, H., Jianchun, Y., Yufeng, Z. and Jianxia, L. (1999). Study on changes of aroma components in flue-cured tobacco during fermentation and aging [J]. *Acta Tabacaria Sinica, 4.*

Daniell, H., Cohill, P. R., Kumar, S. and Dufourmantel, N. (2004). Chloroplast genetic engineering. In *Molecular Biology and Biotechnology of Plant Organelles* (pp. 443-490): Springer.

Daniell, H., Khan, M. S. and Allison, L. (2002). Milestones in chloroplast genetic engineering: an environmentally friendly era in biotechnology. *Trends in Plant Science,* 7(2): 84-91.

Daniell, H., Lin, C. S., Yu, M. and Chang, W. J. (2016). Chloroplast genomes: diversity, evolution, and applications in genetic engineering. *Genome Biology,* 17(1): 134.

Daniell, H., Ruiz, O. N. and Dhingra, A. (2005). Chloroplast genetic engineering to improve agronomic traits. In *Transgenic Plants: Methods and Protocols* (pp. 111-137): Springer.

Daròs, J. A. and Flores, R. (2004). *Arabidopsis thaliana* has the enzymatic machinery for replicating representative viroid species of the family

Pospiviroidae. *Proceedings of the National Academy of Sciences,* 101(17): 6792-6797.

Davis, D. L. and Nielsen, M. T. (1999). *Tobacco: production, chemistry and technology*: Blackwell Science: Oxford, UK.

Demirbas, A., Bafail, A., Ahmad, W. and Sheikh, M. (2016). Biodiesel production from non-edible plant oils. *Energy Exploration & Exploitation,* 34(2): 290-318.

Dickson, S. A. (1954). *Panacea or Precious Bane: Tobacco in 16th Century literature*: Public Libr.

Domino, E. F. (1999). Pharmacological significance of nicotine. *In: J. W. Garrod and P. Jacob III (Editors), Analytical determination of nicotine and related compounds and their metabolites (first ed.)* (pp. 1-12): Elsevier Science B. V., Amstrerdam, The Netherlands.

Erickson, L., Yu, W. J., Brandle, J. and Rymerson, R. (2013). *Molecular farming of plants and animals for human and veterinary medicine*: Springer Science & Business Media.

Eriksen, M., Mackay, J. and Ross, H. (2015). The tobacco atlas. Atlanta, Georgia: American Cancer Society. *Word Lung.*

Eriksen, M., Mackay, J., Schluger, N., Gomeshtapeh, F. and Drope, J. (2015). *The Tobacco Atlas: Revised, Expanded, and Updated.* Atlanta, USA: American Cancer Society, Inc.

Fantozzi, P. and Sensidoni, A. (1983). Protein extraction from tobacco leaves: technological, nutritional and agronomical aspects. *Plant Foods for Human Nutrition,* 32(3): 351-368.

Feinhandler, S. J., Fleming, H. C. and Monahon, J. M. (1979). Pre-Columbian tobaccos in the Pacific. *Economic Botany,* 33(2): 213-226.

Fernandez-Pozo, N., Menda, N., Edwards, J. D., Saha, S., Tecle, I. Y., Strickler, S. R., et al. (2014). The Sol Genomics Network (SGN)-from genotype to phenotype to breeding. *Nucleic Acids Research,* 43(D1): D1036-D1041.

Food and Agriculture Organization of the United Nations (FAOSTAT) (2016). *Crops.* Tobacco, production quantity. http://www.fao.org/faostat/en/.

Fogher, C. (2008). *Mutagenized tobacco plant as seed culture for the production of oil for energetic, industrial and alimentary uses*. Patent application WO/2008/110876.

Fogher, C., Norscia, N. and Tommasini, S. (2011). Developing tobacco's potential as a novel, high-yielding, renewable energy plant. *International News on Fats, Oils and Related Materials,* 22: 631-634.

Fox, J. L. (2006). Turning plants into protein factories. *Nature Biotechnlogy*, 24: 1191-1193.

Fox, J. L. (2011). HIV drugs made in tobacco. *Nature Biotechnology,* 29(10): 852-852.

Frankenburg, W. G. (1946). Chemical changes in the harvested tobacco leaf: part I. Chemical and enzymic conversions during the curing process. *Advances in Enzymology and Related Areas of Molecular Biology,* 6: 309-387.

Franklin, R. E., Caspar, D. L. and Klug, A. (1958). The structure of viruses as determined by X-ray diffraction. *Plant Pathology, Problems and Progress,* 1958: 447-461.

Fulneček, J., Matyášek, R. and Kovařík, A. (2009). Faithful inheritance of cytosine methylation patterns in repeated sequences of the allotetraploid tobacco correlates with the expression of DNA methyltransferase gene families from both parental genomes. *Molecular Genetics and Genomics,* 281(4): 407-420.

Gadani, F., Ayers, D. and Hempfling, W. (1995). Tobacco: a tool for plant genetic engineering research and molecular farming. Part I. *Agro Food Ind. Hi-Tech,* 6: 19-24.

Ganapathi T, P. S., Rao PS, Bapat V (2004). Tobacco (*Nicotiana tabacum* L.) - a model system for tissue culture interventions and genetic engineering. *Indian Journal of Biotechnology,* 3(2): 171-184.

Gao, H. J., Zhang, X. Z., Zhong, J. J., Liu, D. H., Yang, J. and Yin, J. (2011). Research on extraction tobacco essential oils by steam distillation. *Science and Technology of Food Industry,* 10.

Garner, W. (1941). Climate and tobacco. *US Agr. Yearbook*. 1941: 364-372.

Garner, W. W. (1909). *Principles and practical methods of curing tobacco.*

Garner, W. W. (1949). *Tobacco culture* (Vol. No. 571): US Dept. of Agriculture.

Garner, W. W. (1951). The production of tobacco. *McGraw Hill, New York, United States*, 516.

Gazdova, B., Siroky, J., Fajkus, J., Brzobohaty, B., Kenton, A., Parokonny, A., et al. (1995). Characterization of a new family of tobacco highly repetitive DNA, GRS, specific for the *Nicotiana-tomentosiformis* genomic component. *Chromosome Research*, 3(4): 245-254.

Geelen, D. N. and Inzé, D. G. (2001). A bright future for the bright yellow-2 cell culture. *Plant Physiology*, 127(4): 1375-1379.

Gerstel, D. U. (1963). Segregation in new allopolyploids of *Nicotiana* .2. Discordant ratios from individual loci in 6× (*N. tabacum* × *N. sylvestris*). *Genetics*, 48(5): 677-689.

Gill, B. S. and Friebe, B. (2013). Nucleocytoplasmic interaction hypothesis of genome evolution and speciation in polyploid plants revisited: Polyploid species-specific chromosomal polymorphisms in wheat. In: In: Chen ZJ, Birchler JA (eds.) *Polyploid and Hybrid Genomics*. Wiley, New York, 213-221.

Gode, P. (1957). References to tobacco in some Sanskrit works between AD 1600 and 1900. *Annals of the Bhandarkar Oriental Research Institute*, 38(3/4): 225-232.

Goodin, M. M., Zaitlin, D., Naidu, R. A. and Lommel, S. A. (2008). *Nicotiana benthamiana*: its history and future as a model for plant-pathogen interactions. *Molecular Plant-Microbe Interactions*, 21(8): 1015-1026.

Goodman, J. (1993). *Tobacco in history: The cultures of dependence*: London: Routledge.

Goodspeed, T. H. (1954). *The genus Nicotiana* (Vol. 16, Chronica Botanica). Massachusetts, USA: Waltham.

Goodspeed, T. H. (1954). The genus *Nicotiana*: Origins, relationships and evolution of its species in the light of their distribution, morphology and cytogenetics. *Chronica Botanica Company*, Waltham, MA, USA, and Stechert-Hafner, Inc. 1955, New York, NY, USA.

Grant-Downton, R. and Dickinson, H. (2005). Epigenetics and its implications for plant biology. 1. The epigenetic network in plants. *Annals of Botany,* 96(7): 1143-1164.

Grisan, S., Polizzotto, R., Raiola, P., Cristiani, S., Ventura, F., di Lucia, F., et al. (2016). Alternative use of tobacco as a sustainable crop for seed oil, biofuel, and biomass. *Agronomy for Sustainable Development,* 36(4): 55.

Grise, V. N. and Griffin, K. F. (1988). *The US tobacco industry*: US Department of Agriculture, Economic Research Service.

Gullón, P., María Jesús, G. M. and Juan Carlos, P. (2011). Manufacture and prebiotic potential of oligosaccharides derived from industrial solid wastes. *Bioresource Technology,* 102(10): 6112-6119.

Hajdu, S. I. and Vadmal, M. S. (2010). The use of tobacco. *Annals of Clinical & Laboratory Science,* 40(2): 178-181.

Haley, D., Nasset, E. and Olson, O. (1928). A study of certain constituents of the leaf and their relation to the burning qualities of tobacco. *Plant Physiology,* 3(2): 185.

Hanafin, J. and Clancy, L. (2015). History of tobacco production and use. In *The Tobacco Epidemic.* Karger Publishers. 42: 1-18.

Harashima, H., Shinmyo, A. and Sekine, M. (2007). Phosphorylation of threonine 161 in plant cyclin-dependent kinase A is required for cell division by activation of its associated kinase. *The Plant Journal,* 52(3): 435-448.

Hartana, I. and Vermeulen, H. (2016). *Nicotiana tabacum* (PROSEA). https://uses.plantnet-project.org/en/Nicotiana_tabacum_(PROSEA).

Hartmann-Boyce, J., Chepkin, S. C., Ye, W., Bullen, C. and Lancaster, T. (2018). Nicotine replacement therapy versus control for smoking cessation. *Cochrane Database of Systematic Reviews* (5).

Hawks Jr, S. and Collins, W. (1994). Načela proizvodnje virginijskog duhana. *Ceres, Zagreb, 369*. [Principles of Virginia tobacco production. Ceres, Zagreb, 369]

Heslop-Harrison, J. S. and Schwarzacher, T. (2011). Organisation of the plant genome in chromosomes. *Plant Journal,* 66(1): 18-33.

Hibi, N., Higashiguchi, S., Hashimoto, T. and Yamada, Y. (1994). Gene-Expression in tobacco low-nicotine mutants. *Plant Cell,* 6(5): 723-735.

Hirochika, H. (1993). Activation of tobacco retrotransposons during tissue-culture. *EMBO Journal,* 12(6): 2521-2528.

Hoekema, A., Hirsch, P. R., Hooykaas, P. J. and Schilperoort, R. A. (1983). A binary plant vector strategy based on separation of vir-and T-region of the *Agrobacterium tumefaciens* Ti-plasmid. *Nature,* 303(5913): 179.

Holtz, B. R., Berquist, B. R., Bennett, L. D., Kommineni, V. J., Munigunti, R. K., White, E. L., et al. (2015). Commercial-scale biotherapeutics manufacturing facility for plant-made pharmaceuticals. *Plant Biotechnology Journal,* 13(8): 1180-1190.

Horn, M., Woodard, S. and Howard, J. (2004). Plant molecular farming: systems and products. *Plant cell reports,* 22(10): 711-720.

Hughes, J. R. (2000). Nicotine related disorders. In*: Sadock, Benjamin J, Sadock, Virginia A. Kaplan & Sadock's Concise Textbook of Clinical Psychiatry*: 7. Philadelphia, Lippincott: Williams & Wilkins.

International Labour Organization (ILO) (2003). *ILO: Up in smoke: What future for tobacco jobs?* https://www.ilo.org/global/about-the-ilo/newsroom/features/WCMS_071230/lang--en/index.htm.

Iqbal, Z., Lateef, M., Jabbar, A., Ghayur, M. N. and Gilani, A. H. (2006). *In vitro* and *in vivo* anthelmintic activity of *Nicotiana tabacum* L. leaves against gastrointestinal nematodes of sheep. *Phytotherapy Research: An International Journal Devoted to Pharmacological and Toxicological Evaluation of Natural Product Derivatives,* 20(1): 46-48.

Iriti, M., Kubina, R., Cochis, A., Sorrentino, R., Varoni, E. M., Kaba-Dzik, A., et al. (2017). Rutin, a quercetin glycoside, restores chemosensitivity in human breast cancer cells. *Phytotherapy Research,* 31(10): 1529-1538.

Jakowitsch, J., Papp, I., Matzke, M. A. and Matzke, A. J. M. (1998). Identification of a new family of highly repetitive DNA, NTS9, that is located predominantly on the S9 chromosome of tobacco. *Chromosome Research,* 6(8): 649-651.

James, C. (2001). *Global Review of Commercialized Transgenic Crops. ISAAA Briefs No. 24*: Preview. Ithaca, NY: International Service for the

Acquisition of Agri-Biotech Applications. (http://www.isaaa.org/publications/briefs/Brief_24.htm).

Jeffrey, R. and Tso, T. (1955). Tobacco constituents, qualitative differences in alkaloid fraction of cured tobaccos. *Journal of Agricultural and Food Chemistry,* 3(8): 680-682.

Johnson, P. R. (1984). *The economics of the tobacco industry*: Praeger, New York, NY, USA.

Joshi, M. (2018). Rabi commercial crops. Part 12. Tobacco (*Nicotiana tabacum* L.). *Textbook of field crops*. PHI Learning Pvt. Ltd.

Jube, S. and Borthakur, D. (2007). Expression of bacterial genes in transgenic tobacco: methods, applications and future prospects. *Electronic Journal of Biotechnology,* 10(3): 452-467.

Kajikawa, M., Sierro, N., Hashimoto, T. and Shoji, T. (2017a). A model for evolution and regulation of nicotine biosynthesis regulon in tobacco. *Plant Signaling & Behavior,* 12(6): e1338225.

Kajikawa, M., Sierro, N., Kawaguchi, H., Bakaher, N., Ivanov, N. V., Hashimoto, T., et al. (2017b). Genomic insights into the evolution of the nicotine biosynthesis pathway in tobacco. *Plant Physiology,* 174(2): 999-1011.

Kaldis, A., Ahmad, A., Reid, A., McGarvey, B., Brandle, J., Ma, S., et al. (2013). High-level production of human interleukin-10 fusions in tobacco cell suspension cultures. *Plant Biotechnology Journal,* 11(5): 535-545.

Keinänen, M., Oldham, N. J. and Baldwin, I. T. (2001). Rapid HPLC screening of jasmonate-induced increases in tobacco alkaloids, phenolics, and diterpene glycosides in *Nicotiana attenuata*. *Journal of Agricultural and Food Chemistry,* 49(8): 3553-3558.

Kenton, A., Parokonny, A. S., Gleba, Y. Y. and Bennett, M. D. (1993). Characterization of the *Nicotiana tabacum* L. genome by molecular cytogenetics. *Molecular and General Genetics,* 240(2): 159-169.

Kessler, D., Diezel, C. and Baldwin, I. T. (2010). Changing pollinators as a means of escaping herbivores. *Current Biology,* 20(3): 237-242.

Kim, H. J., Yano, A., Wada, Y. and Sano, H. (2007). Properties of a tobacco DNA methyltransferase, *NtMET1* and its involvement in chromatin movement during cell division. *Annals of Botany,* 99(5): 845-856.

Kishore, K. (2014). Monograph of tobacco (*Nicotiana tabacum*). *Indian Journal of Drugs,* 2(1): 5-23.

Klein, T. M., Harper, E. C., Svab, Z., Sanford, J. C., Fromm, M. E. and Maliga, P. (1988). Stable genetic transformation of intact *Nicotiana* cells by the particle bombardment process. *Proceedings of the National Academy of Sciences,* 85(22): 8502-8505.

Knapp, S., Chase, M. W. and Clarkson, J. J. (2004). Nomenclatural changes and a new sectional classification in *Nicotiana* (Solanaceae). *Taxon,* 53(1): 73-82.

Koornneef, M. and Meinke, D. (2010). The development of *Arabidopsis* as a model plant. *The Plant Journal,* 61(6): 909-921.

Koukalova, B., Fojtova, M., Lim, K. Y., Fulnecek, J., Leitch, A. R. and Kovarik, A. (2005). Dedifferentiation of tobacco cells is associated with ribosomal RNA gene hypomethylation, increased transcription, and chromatin alterations. *Plant Physiology,* 139(1): 275-286.

Koukalova, B., Kovarik, A., Fajkus, J. and Siroky, J. (1997). Chromatin fragmentation associated with apoptotic changes in tobacco cells exposed to cold stress. *FEBS Letters,* 414(2): 289-292.

Koukalova, B., Moraes, A. P., Renny-Byfield, S., Matyasek, R., Leitch, A. R. and Kovarik, A. (2010). Fall and rise of satellite repeats in allopolyploids of *Nicotiana* over c. 5 million years. *New Phytologist,* 186(1): 148-160.

Koukalova, B., Reich, J., Matyášek, R., Kuhrova, V. and Bezděk, M. (1989). A BamHI family of highly repeated DNA sequences of *Nicotiana tabacum*. *Theoretical and Applied Genetics,* 78: 77-80.

Kovarik, A., Koukalova, B., Bezdek, M. and Opatrny, Z. (1997). Hypermethylation of tobacco heterochromatic loci in response to osmotic stress. *Theoretical and Applied Genetics,* 95(1-2): 301-306.

Křížová, K., Depicker, A. and Kovařík, A. (2013). Epigenetic switches of tobacco transgenes associate with transient redistribution of histone marks in callus culture. *Epigenetics,* 8(6): 666-676.

Kuehn, B. M. (2006). FDA speeds smoking cessation drug review. *Jama,* 295(6): 614-614.

Kung, S. D. (1976). Tobacco fraction 1 protein: a unique genetic marker. *Science,* 191(4226): 429-434.

Kung, S., Saunder, J. A., Tso, T., Vaughan, D. A., Womack, M., Staples, R. C., et al. (1980). Tobacco as a potential food source and smoke material: nutritional evaluation of tobacco leaf protein. *Journal of Food Science,* 45(2): 320-322.

Kung, S. and Tso, T. (1978). Tobacco as a potential food source and smoke material: soluble protein content, extraction, and amino acid composition. *Journal of Food Science,* 43(6): 1844-1847.

Kuthanova, A., Fischer, L., Nick, P. and Opatrny, Z. (2008). Cell cycle phase-specific death response of tobacco BY-2 cell line to cadmium treatment. *Plant, Cell & Environment,* 31(11): 1634-1643.

Kutik, J., Kuthanova, A., Smertenko, A., Fischer, L. and Opatrny, Z. (2014). Cadmium-induced cell death in BY-2 cell culture starts with vacuolization of cytoplasm and terminates with necrosis. *Physiologia Plantarum,* 151(4): 423-433.

Lal, C. and Verma, L. (2006). Use of certain bio-products for insect-pest control. *Indian Journal of Traditional Knowledge,* 5(1): 79-82.

Langer, R. H. M. and Hill, G. (1991). *Agricultural plants*: Cambridge University Press.

Langreth, R., Chen, C., Nash, J. and Lauerman, J. (2014). Ebola drug made from tobacco plant saves US aid workers. *Bloomberg.com.*

Larrick, J., Yu, L., Chen, J., Jaiswal, S. and Wycoff, K. (1998). Production of antibodies in transgenic plants. *Research in Immunology,* 149(6): 603-608.

Laws, B. (2010). *Fifty plants that changed the course of history*: Firefly Books Ltd.

Lewis, R. and Nicholson, J. (2007). Aspects of the evolution of *Nicotiana tabacum* L. and the status of the United States *Nicotiana* germplasm collection. *Genetic Resources and Crop Evolution,* 54(4): 727-740.

Lim, K. Y., Matyasek, R., Kovarik, A. and Leitch, A. R. (2004a). Genome evolution in allotetraploid *Nicotiana. Biological Journal of the Linnean Society,* 82(4): 599-606.

Lim, K. Y., Skalicka, K., Koukalova, B., Volkov, R. A., Matyasek, R., Hemleben, V., et al. (2004b). Dynamic changes in the distribution of a satellite homologous to intergenic 26-18S rDNA spacer in the evolution of *Nicotiana. Genetics*, 166(4): 1935-1946.

Lin, Y. T., Wei, H. M., Lu, H. Y., Lee, Y. I. and Fu, S. F. (2015). Developmental-and tissue-specific expression of *NbCMT3-2* encoding a chromomethylase in *Nicotiana benthamiana. Plant and Cell Physiology,* 56(6): 1124-1143.

Liu, B. and Wendel, J. F. (2003). Epigenetic phenomena and the evolution of plant allopolyploids. *Molecular Phylogenetics and Evolution,* 29(3): 365-379.

Liu, X. and Zhang, H. (2008). Advance of molecular marker application in the tobacco research. *African Journal of Biotechnology,* 7(25).

Lonitzer, A. and Uffenbach, P. K. (1630). *The Bavarian State Library*.

Luthra, U. K., Sreeniva, V., Menon, G., Prabhakar, A. and Chaudhry, K. Tobacco control in India: Problems and solutions. In *Control of Tobacco-related Cancers and Other Diseases: Proceedings of an International Symposium, January 15-19, 1990, TIFR, Bombay, 1992* (pp. 241): Prakash C. Gupta.

Ma, J., Drake, P. and Christou, P. (2003). The production of recombinant pharmaceutical proteins in plants. *Nature reviews. Genetics,* 4: 794-805.

Ma, J. K. C., Drossard, J., Lewis, D., Altmann, F., Boyle, J., Christou, P., et al. (2015). Regulatory approval and a first-in human phase I clinical trial of a monoclonal antibody produced in transgenic tobacco plants. *Plant Biotechnology Journal,* 13(8): 1106-1120.

Manoharlal, R., Saiprasad, G. and Kaikala, V. (2019). Gibberellin A_3 mediated decreased transcriptional rate, mRNA stability and non-competitive inhibition of DNA methyltransferases in tobacco. *Biologia Plantarum,* 63(1): 343-353.

Manoharlal, R., Saiprasad, G., Kaikala, V., Kumar, R. S. and Kovařík, A. (2018a). Analysis of DNA methylome and transcriptome profiling following gibberellin A_3 (GA_3) foliar application in *Nicotiana tabacum* L. *Indian Journal of Plant Physiology,* 23(3): 543-556.

Manoharlal, R., Saiprasad, G., Ullagaddi, C. and Kovařík, A. (2018b). Gibberellin A_3 as an epigenetic determinant of global DNA hypomethylation in tobacco. *Biologia Plantarum,* 62(1): 11-23.

Matyasek, R., Gazdova, B., Fajkus, J. and Bezdek, M. (1997). NTRS, a new family of highly repetitive DNAs specific for the T1 chromosome of tobacco. *Chromosoma,* 106(6): 369-379.

Matzke, M., Gregor, W., Mette, M. F., Aufsatz, W., Kanno, T., Jakowitsch, J., et al. (2004). Endogenous pararetroviruses of allotetraploid *Nicotiana tabacum* and its diploid progenitors, *N. sylvestris* and *N. tomentosiformis*. *Biological Journal of the Linnean Society,* 82(4): 627-638.

Mayne, R. G. (1860). *An expository lexicon of the terms, ancient and modern, in medical and general science: Including a complete medico-legal vocabulary, and presenting the correct pronunciation, derivation... of the names, analogues... connected with medicine and employed in the natural sciences*: John Churchill.

McCants, C. and Woltz, W. (1967). Growth and mineral nutrition of tobacco. In *Advances in agronomy*. 19: 211-265.

Meyer, P. (2005). *Plant Epigenetics*: Oxford: Blackwell Publication.

Mhazo, M. L., Mhazo, N. and Masarirambi, M. T. (2011). The effectiveness of home made organic pesticides derived from wild plants (*Solanum pindiriforme* and *Lippia javanica*), garlic (*Allium sativum*) and tobacco (*Nicotiana tobacum*) on aphid (*Brevicoryne brassica*) mortality on rape (*Brassica napus*) plants. *Research Journal of Environmental and Earth Sciences,* 3(5): 457-462.

Miki, B., Mcttugh, S., Labbe, H., Ouellet, T., Tolman, J. and Brandle, J. (1999). Transgenic tobacco: gene expression and applications. In *Transgenic Medicinal Plants* (pp. 336-354): Springer.

Monardes, N. (1970). *Joyfull newes out of the newe founde worlde.* London 1577: W. Norton.

Moscone, E. A., Matzke, M. A. and Matzke, A. J. (1996). The use of combined FISH/GISH in conjunction with DAPI counterstaining to identify chromosomes containing transgene inserts in amphidiploid tobacco. *Chromosoma,* 105(5): 231-236.

Motherby, G. (1791). *A new medical dictionary: Or, general repository of physic. containing an explanation of the terms, and a description of the various particulars relating to anatomy, physiology, physic, surgery, materia medica, chemistry andc. &c. &c. each article, according to its importance, being considered in every relation to which its usefulness extends in the healing art. By G. Motherby, MDCMS by George Wallis, MDSMS lecturer on the theory and practice of physic, London*: J. Johnson, St. Paul's Church-Yard; GGJ and J. Robinson, Paternoster-Row; A. Hamilton, jun. and J. Murray, Fleet-Street.

Mowery, P. D., Dube, S. R., Thorne, S. L., Garrett, B. E., Homa, D. M. and Henderson, P. N. (2015). Disparities in smoking-related mortality among American Indians/Alaska Natives. *American Journal of Preventive Medicine,* 49(5): 738-744.

Mueller, L. A., Solow, T. H., Taylor, N., Skwarecki, B., Buels, R., Binns, J., et al. (2005). The SOL Genomics Network. A comparative resource for Solanaceae biology and beyond. *Plant Physiology,* 138(3): 1310-1317.

Murad, L., Lim, K. Y., Christopodulou, V., Matyasek, R., Lichtenstein, C. P., Kovarik, A., et al. (2002). The origin of tobacco's T genome is traced to a particular lineage within *Nicotiana tomentosiformis* (Solanaceae). *American Journal of Botany,* 89(6): 921-928.

Murashige, T. and Skoog, F. (1962). A revised medium for rapid growth and bio assays with tobacco tissue cultures. *Physiologia Plantarum,* 15(3): 473-497.

Nadkarni, K. M. (1996). *[Indian materia medica]; Dr. KM Nadkarni's Indian materia medica: with Ayurvedic, Unani-Tibbi, Siddha, allopathic, homeopathic, naturopathic & home remedies, appendices & indexes. 1* (Vol. 1): Popular Prakashan.

Nagaki, K., Shibata, F. and Murata, M. (2011). A mosaic structure of centromeric DNA in tobacco. *Genes & Genetic Systems,* 86(6): 434-434.

Nagata, T., Nemoto, Y. and Hasezawa, S. (1992). Tobacco BY-2 cell line as the "HeLa" cell in the cell biology of higher plants. *International Review of Cytology*, 132: 1-30.

Nagata, T. and Takebe, I. (1971). Plating of isolated tobacco mesophyll protoplasts on agar medium. *Planta,* 99(1): 12-20.

Nair, N. R., Chidambareswaren, M. and Manjula, S. (2014). Enhanced heterologous expression of biologically active human granulocyte colony stimulating factor in transgenic tobacco BY-2 cells by localization to endoplasmic reticulum. *Molecular Biotechnology,* 56(9): 849-862.

Nakano, Y., Steward, N., Sekine, M., Kusano, T. and Sano, H. (2000). A tobacco *NtMET1* cDNA encoding a DNA methyltransferase: molecular characterization and abnormal phenotypes of transgenic tobacco plants. *Plant and Cell Physiology,* 41(4): 448-457.

Nitsch, J. and Ohyama, K. (1971). Obtention de plantes à partir de protoplastes haploïdes cultivés in vitro. *Acad Sci Paris CR Ser D.* 273: 801-804. [Obtaining plants from haploid protoplasts grown in vitro. *Comptes rendus de l'Académie des Sciences.* 273: 801-804.].

Nocarova, E. and Fischer, L. (2009). Cloning of transgenic tobacco BY-2 cells; an efficient method to analyse and reduce high natural heterogeneity of transgene expression. *BMC Plant Biology,* 9(1): 44.

Nouri, F., Nourollahi-Fard, S. R., Foroodi, H. R. and Sharifi, H. (2016). *In vitro* anthelmintic effect of tobacco (*Nicotiana tabacum*) extract on parasitic nematode, *Marshallagia marshalli. Journal of parasitic diseases: Official organ of the Indian Society for Parasitology,* 40(3): 643-647.

Ogura, H. (1976). The cytological chimeras in original regenerates from tobacco tissue cultures and in their offsprings. *The Japanese Journal of Genetics,* 51(3): 161-174.

Okamuro, J. K. and Goldberg, R. B. (1985). Tobacco single-copy DNA is highly homologous to sequences present in the genomes of its diploid progenitors. *Molecular and General Genetics,* 198(2): 290-298.

Olmstead, R. G., Bohs, L., Migid, H. A., Santiago-Valentin, E., Garcia, V. F. and Collier, S. M. (2008). A molecular phylogeny of the Solanaceae. *Taxon,* 57(4): 1159-1181.

Paul, M., Dolleweerd, C. v., Drake, P. M. W., Reljic, R., Thangaraj, H., Barbi, T., et al. (2011). Molecular pharming. *Human Vaccines,* 7(3): 375-382.

Peedin, G. F. (2002). Tobacco cultivation. In: *Specialty crops* (ed. Myers M. L. International Labor Organization).

Petit, M., Guidat, C., Daniel, J., Denis, E., Montoriol, E., Bui, Q. T., et al. (2010). Mobilization of retrotransposons in synthetic allotetraploid tobacco. *New Phytologist,* 186(1): 135-147.

Petit, M., Lim, K. Y., Julio, E., Poncet, C., Dorlhac de Borne, F., Kovarik, A., et al. (2007). Differential impact of retrotransposon populations on the genome of allotetraploid tobacco (*Nicotiana tabacum*). *Molecular Genetics and Genomics,* 278(1): 1-15.

PFAF (2014). *Plants for a future.* http://www.pfaf.org.

Pomerleau, O. F. and Pomerleau, C. S. (1991). Research on stress and smoking: progress and problems. *British Journal of Addiction,* 86(5): 599-603.

Posselt, W. and Reimann, L. (1828). Chemische Untersuchungen des Tabaks und Darstellung des eigenhumlichen wirksamen Principes dieser Pflanze. *Geigers Magazin der Pharmazie,* 24: 138-161. [Chemical examinations of the tobacco and presentation of the intrinsically effective principle of this plant. *Geiger's Pharmacy Magazine*, 24: 138-161].

Pouteau, S., Huttner, E., Grandbastien, M. A. and Caboche, M. (1991). Specific expression of the tobacco Tnt1 retrotransposon in protoplasts. *EMBO Journal,* 10(7): 1911-1918.

Puripattanavong, J., Songkram, C., Lomlim, L. and Amnuaikit, T. (2013). Development of concentrated emulsion containing *Nicotiana tabacum* extract for use as pesticide. *Journal of Applied Pharmaceutical Science,* 3(11): 16.

Randall, R. (2012). *A Global Compendium of Weeds.* Perth, Australia: Department of Agriculture and Food Western Australia, 1124 pp.

Rao, S. V., Narasimha Rao, C. V. and Deo Singh, K. (2005). Bioengineered products from tobacco: Alternative uses of tobacco. Deo Singh K and

Jain KC (Eds). *Central Tobacco Research Institute, Rajahmundry,* India, 116-134.

Ren, N. and Timko, M. P. (2001). AFLP analysis of genetic polymorphism and evolutionary relationships among cultivated and wild *Nicotiana* species. *Genome,* 44(4): 559-571.

Renny-Byfield, S., Chester, M., Kovařík, A., S. C., L. C., Grandbastien, M. A., M., D., et al. (2011). Next generation sequencing reveals evidence of genome downsizing and elimination of paternally derived repetitive DNA sequences in tobacco. *Molecular Biology and Evolution,* 28(10): 2843-2854.

Renny-Byfield, S., Kovarik, A., Chester, M., Nichols, R. A., Macas, J., Novak, P., et al. (2012). Independent, rapid and targeted loss of highly repetitive DNA in natural and synthetic allopolyploids of *Nicotiana tabacum. PLoS ONE,* 7(5): e36963.

Řepková, J. (2010). Potential of chloroplast genome in plant breeding. *Czech Journal of Genetics and Plant Breeding,* 46(3): 103-113.

ResearchAndMarkets.com (2017). *Tobacco market global briefing 2018-Global tobacco market 2018: Historic analysis and forecasts* (2013-2021). https://www.researchandmarkets.com/research/7wgjpv/global_tobacco?w=4.

ResearchAndMarkets.com (2019). *Cigarette market: Global industry trends, share, size, growth, opportunity and forecast* 2019-2024. https://www.researchandmarkets.com/research/qj2jd5/global_cigarette?w=5.

Rossi, L., Fusi, E., Baldi, G., Fogher, C., Cheli, F., Baldi, A., et al. (2013). Tobacco seeds by-product as protein source for piglets. *Open Journal of Veterinary Medicine,* 3(01): 73.

Roumeli, E., Bonanomi, L., Hendrickx, R., Rinaldi, K. and Daraio, C. (2019). Plant cells-based biological matrix composites. *arXiv preprint arXiv:1909.01926.*

Rowland, R. L., Latimer, P. and Giles, J. (1956). Flue-cured tobacco. I. Isolation of solanesol, an unsaturated alcohol. *Journal of the American Chemical Society,* 78(18): 4680-4683.

Rufty, R., Wernsman, E. and Gooding Jr, G. (1988). Inheritance of tobacco etch virus resistance found in *Nicotiana tabacum* cultivar Havana 307. *Plant Disease (USA)*.

Rushton, P. J., Bokowiec, M. T., Han, S., Zhang, H., Brannock, J. F., Chen, X., et al. (2008). Tobacco transcription factors: novel insights into transcriptional regulation in the Solanaceae. *Plant Physiology,* 147(1): 280-295.

Russo, P., Cesario, A., Rutella, S., Veronesi, G., Spaggiari, L., Galetta, D., et al. (2011). Impact of genetic variability in nicotinic acetylcholine receptors on nicotine addiction and smoking cessation treatment. *Current Medicinal Chemistry,* 18(1): 91-112.

Rymerson, R. T., Menassa, R. and Brandle, J. E. (2002). Tobacco, a platform for the production of recombinant proteins. In L. Erickson, W. J. Yu, J. Brandle and R. Rymerson (Eds.), *Molecular Farming of Plants and Animals for Human and Veterinary Medicine* (pp. 1-31). Dordrecht: Springer Netherlands.

Salmon, E. J. and Salmon, J. (2013). Tobacco in Colonial Virginia. *Encyclopedia Virginia.* Virginia Foundation for the Humanities. Retrieved August, 19, 2013.

Sarala, K., Murthy, T., Prabhakara Rao, K. and Ravisankar, H. (2013). Tobacco Research in India: Trends and Developments. *Agrotechnology,* 2(3): 113.

Schaeffer, S., Koepke, T. and Dhingra, A. (2012). Tobacco: A model plant for understanding the mechanism of abiotic stress tolerance. In *In improving crop resistance to abiotic stress* (eds N. Tuteja, S. S. Gill, A. F. Tiburcio and R. Tuteja*)* (pp. 1169-1201).

Schmitt, F., Oakeley, E. J. and Jost, J. P. (1997). Antibiotics induce genome-wide hypermethylation in cultured *Nicotiana tabacum* plants. *Journal of Biological Chemistry,* 272(3): 1534-1540.

Shakhes, J., Marandi, M. A., Zeinaly, F., Saraian, A. and Saghafi, T. (2011). Tobacco residuals as promising lignocellulosic materials for pulp and paper industry. *BioResources,* 6(4): 4481-4493.

Sheen, S. J. and Sheen, V. L. (1985). Functional properties of fraction 1 protein from tobacco leaf. *Journal of Agricultural and Food Chemistry,* 33(1): 79-83.

Shibata, F., Nagaki, K., Yokota, E. and Murata, M. (2013). Tobacco karyotyping by accurate centromere identification and novel repetitive DNA localization. *Chromosome Research,* 21(4): 375-381.

Shinozaki, K., Ohme, M., Tanaka, M., Wakasugi, T., Hayashida, N., Matsubayashi, T., et al. (1986). The complete nucleotide sequence of the tobacco chloroplast genome: its gene organization and expression. *EMBO Journal,* 5(9): 2043-2049.

Sierro, N., Battey, J. N., Ouadi, S., Bakaher, N., Bovet, L., Willig, A., et al. (2014). The tobacco genome sequence and its comparison with those of tomato and potato. *Nature Communications,* 5: 3833.

Sierro, N., Battey, J. N., Ouadi, S., Bovet, L., Goepfert, S., Bakaher, N., et al. (2013). Reference genomes and transcriptomes of *Nicotiana sylvestris* and *Nicotiana tomentosiformis*. *Genome Biology,* 14(6): R60.

Sijmons, P. C., Dekker, B. M., Schrammeijer, B., Verwoerd, T. C., Van Den Elzen, P. J. and Hoekema, A. (1990). Production of correctly processed human serum albumin in transgenic plants. *Biotechnology,* 8(3): 217.

Siminszky, B., Chakrabarti, M., Meekins, K. M. and Gavilano, L. B. (2007). Inactivation of the cytochrome P450 gene *CYP82E2* by degenerative mutations was a key event in the evolution of the alkaloid profile of modern tobacco. *New Phytologist,* 175(3): 565-574.

Skalicka, K., Lim, K. Y., Matyasek, R., Matzke, M., Leitch, A. R. and Kovarik, A. (2005). Preferential elimination of repeated DNA sequences from the paternal, *Nicotiana tomentosiformis* genome donor of a synthetic, allotetraploid tobacco. *New Phytologist,* 166(1): 291-303.

Skoog, F. and Miller, C. (1957). Chemical regulation of growth and organ formation in plant tissues cultured. In *Vitro, Symposia of the Society for Experimental Biology,* No. 11.

Smykal, P., Gleissner, R., Corbesier, L., Apel, K. and Melzer, S. (2004). Modulation of flowering responses in different *Nicotiana* varieties. *Plant Molecular Biology,* 55(2): 253-262.

Spiegel, H., Stöger, E., Twyman, R. M. and Buyel, J. F. (2018). Current status and perspectives of the molecular farming landscape. *Molecular Pharming: Applications, Challenges and Emerging Areas*, 3-23.

Srivastava, S., Raj, K., Khare, P., Bhaduri, A. P., Chander, R., Raghubir, R., et al. (2009). Novel hybrid natural products derived from solanesol as wound healing agents. *Indian Journal of Chemistry,* 48: 1-12.

Stanisavljević, I., Svetlana Lakićević, Dragan Veličković, Miodrag Lazić and Veljković, V. (2007). The extraction of oil from tobacco (*Nicotiana tabacum* L.) seeds. *Chemical Industry and Chemical Engineering Quarterly/CICEQ,* 13(1): 41-50.

Stanley, W. M. (1935). Isolation of a crystalline protein possessing the properties of tobacco-mosaic virus. *Science,* 81(2113): 644-645.

States, U. (1989). U.S. Department of Agriculture, Marketing & Regulatory Programs, Agricultural Marketing Service, Tobacco Programs 1989. *Official standard grades for flue-cured tobacco: U.S. types 11, 12, 13, 14 and foreign type 92: Effective* March 27, 1989 (54 F. R. 7925). U.S. Government Printing Office (U. S. GPO). Washington, DC. (*Agriculture Marketing Series*).

Steinberg, R. A. and Tso, T. C. (1958). Physiology of the tobacco plant. *Annual Review of Plant Physiology,* 9(1): 151-174.

Stewart, G. G. (1967). A history of the medicinal use of tobacco 1492-1860. *Medical History,* 11(3): 228-268.

Sussex, I. M. (2008). The scientific roots of modern plant biotechnology. *The Plant Cell,* 20(5): 1189-1198.

Sutherland, J. E. and Costa, M. (2003). Epigenetics and the environment. *Annals of the New York Academy of Sciences,* 983(1): 151-160.

Takahashi, S., Kojo, K. H., Kutsuna, N., Endo, M., Toki, S., Lsoda, H., et al. (2015). Differential responses to high- and low-dose ultraviolet-B stress in tobacco Bright Yellow-2 cells. *Frontiers in Plant Science,* 6:254.

Talhout, R., Schulz, T., Florek, E., Van Benthem, J., Wester, P. and Opperhuizen, A. (2011). Hazardous compounds in tobacco smoke. *International Journal of Environmental Research and Public Health,* 8(2): 613-628.

Tao, Z. and Shudong, Z. (2003). The economic and social impact of GMOs in China. *China Perspectives, 2003*(47).

Technology Information, F. A. C., New Delhi (2004). *Nicotine and its derivatives from tobacco waste.* https://tifac.org.in/index.php/8-publication/192-nicotine-and-its-derivatives-from-tobacco-waste.

Tiwari, S., Verma, P. C., Singh, P. K. and Tuli, R. (2009). Plants as bioreactors for the production of vaccine antigens. *Biotechnology Advances,* 27(4): 449-467.

Tong, Z., Xiao, B., Jiao, F., Fang, D., Zeng, J., Wu, X., et al. (2016). Large-scale development of SSR markers in tobacco and construction of a linkage map in flue-cured tobacco. *Breeding Science,* 66(3): 381-390.

Tong, Z., Yang, Z., Chen, X., Jiao, F., Li, X., Wu, X., et al. (2012). Large-scale development of microsatellite markers in *Nicotiana tabacum* and construction of a genetic map of flue-cured tobacco. *Plant Breeding,* 131(5): 674-680.

Tso, T. C. (1990). *Production, physiology, and biochemistry of tobacco plant*: Ideals.

Tso, T. (2006). Tobacco research and its relevance to science, medicine and industry. *Beiträge zur Tabakforschung International/Contributions to Tobacco Research,* 22(3): 133-145.

Tso, T. and Kung, S. (1983). *Soluble proteins in tobacco and their potential use* (Vol. 117): AVI Publishers, Westport, CT.

USDA: *National Plant Germplasm System*; available at https://www.ars-grin.gov/npgs/. (Accessed August, 2019).

Usman, M. R. M. (2016). *Poisonous herbal plants: NA*: Educreation Publishing.

Van Liemt, G. (2001). *The world tobacco industry: Trends and Prospects*: ILO.

Vanhercke, T., El Tahchy, A., Liu, Q., Zhou, X. R., Shrestha, P., Divi, U. K., et al. (2014). Metabolic engineering of biomass for high energy density: oilseed-like triacylglycerol yields from plant leaves. *Plant Biotechnology Journal,* 12(2): 231-239.

Vasil, V. and Hildebrandt, A. (1965). Differentiation of tobacco plants from single, isolated cells in microcultures. *Science,* 150(3698): 889-892.

Veljković VB, Lakićević SH, Stamenković OS, Todorović ZB and ML, L. (2006). Biodiesel production from tobacco (*Nicotiana tabacum* L.) seed oil with a high content of free fatty acids. *Fuel,* 85(17-18): 2671-2675.

Volkov, R. A., Borisjuk, N. V., Panchuk, II, Schweizer, D. and Hemleben, V. (1999). Elimination and rearrangement of parental rDNA in the allotetraploid *Nicotiana tabacum. Molecular Biology and Evolution,* 16(3): 311-320.

von Linné, C. (1788). *Allgemeines Register über die in den sämtlichen dreyzen Theilen des Linneischen Pflanzensystems beschriebenen Gattungen und Arten nebst einem besondern die denselben eigenen Synonymen erläuternden: Vierzehnter Theil* (Vol. 24): in der Raspischen Buchhandlung. [*General Register of the genera and species described in all the three parts of the Linneian system of plants, together with a special explanation of their own synonyms: The Fourteenth Part* (Vol. 24): in the Raspish Bookstore].

Wada, Y., Ohya, H., Yamaguchi, Y., Koizumi, N. and Sano, H. (2003). Preferential de novo methylation of cytosine residues in non-CpG sequences by a domains rearranged DNA methyltransferase from tobacco plants. *Journal of Biological Chemistry,* 278(43): 42386-42393.

Wang, C., Wang, C., Xu, W., Zou, J., Qiu, Y., Kong, J., et al. (2018). Epigenetic changes in the regulation of *Nicotiana tabacum* response to Cucumber mosaic virus infection and symptom recovery through single-base resolution methylomes. *Viruses,* 10(8): 402.

Wang, Q., Du, H., Zhang, F., Zhang, Y., Wu, M., Yu, G., et al. (2018). Flexible cellulose nanopaper with high wet tensile strength, high toughness and tunable ultraviolet blocking ability fabricated from tobacco stalk via a sustainable method. *Journal of Materials Chemistry A,* 6(27): 13021-13030.

Wasanapiarnpong, T., Nilpairach, S., Siraleartmukul, K., Charoenvai, O., Aungatichart, O. and Laoharungpisit N. (2015). Fabrication of fiber cement using tobacco stalk pulp from agricultural residue. In *Key Engineering Materials,* 659: 102-105. Trans Tech Publications.

Wateson, G. (1915*). The cures of the diseased in forraine attempts of the English nation London, 1598*. Reproduced in facsimile. Clarendon Press.

West, R., Ussher, M., Evans, M. and Rashid, M. (2006). Assessing DSM-IV nicotine withdrawal symptoms: a comparison and evaluation of five different scales. *Psychopharmacology,* 184(3-4): 619-627.

Wildman, S. (1983). An alternate use for tobacco agriculture: proteins for food plus a safer smoking material. In *Plants: The potentials for extracting protein, medicines, and other useful chemicals; Office of Technology Assessment (OTA-BP-F-23):* Washington, DC, USA, 63-67.

Winter, J. C. (2000). Food of the gods: Biochemistry, addiction, and the development of Native American tobacco use. *Tobacco use by Native North Americans: Sacred Smoke and Silent Killer*, 305-330.

Wipfli, H. and Samet, J. M. (2016). One hundred years in the making: the global tobacco epidemic. *Annual Review of Public Health,* 37: 149-166.

Wroblewski, T., Tomczak, A. and Michelmore, R. (2005). Optimization of *Agrobacterium*-mediated transient assays of gene expression in lettuce, tomato and *Arabidopsis*. *Plant Biotechnology Journal,* 3(2): 259-273.

Yan, N., Liu, Y., Gong, D., Du, Y., Zhang, H. and Zhang, Z. (2015). Solanesol: A review of its resources, derivatives, bioactivities, medicinal applications, and biosynthesis. *Phytochemistry Reviews,* 14(3): 403-417.

Yang, B. C., Xiao, B. G., Chen, X. J. and Shi, C. H. (2007). Assessing the genetic diversity of tobacco germplasm using intersimple sequence repeat and inter-retrotransposon amplification polymorphism markers. *Annals of Applied Biology,* 150(3): 393-401.

Yudov, M. (2018). *Tobacco in perfumery: History & chemistry*. https://www.fragrantica.com/news/Tobacco-in-Perfumery-History-Chemistry-11589.html.

Zafeiridou, M., Hopkinson, N. S. and Voulvoulis, N. (2018). Cigarette Smoking: An assessment of tobacco-global environmental footprint across its entire supply chain. *Environmental Science & Technology,* 52(15): 8087-8094.

Zargari, A. (1992). Medicinal plants. *Tehran University Publications, 5th edition,* 3: 889.

Zdremtan, M. and Zdremtan, D. (2006). The tobacco oil and its qualities. *Bulletin USAMV-CN,* 63: 209-213.

Zhang, X., Gao, H., Zhang, L., Liu, D. and Ye, X. (2012). Extraction of essential oil from discarded tobacco leaves by solvent extraction and steam distillation, and identification of its chemical composition. *Industrial Crops and Products,* 39: 162-169.

In: New Research on Tobacco
Editor: Uta Dreher
ISBN: 978-1-53617-077-1

Chapter 3

ELECTRONIC NICOTINE DELIVERY SYSTEMS

Ryan John Pacheco**, DDS, MS
Cochrane Plaza Dental Care, Morgan Hill, CA, US

ABSTRACT

Electronic nicotine delivery system (ENDS), also known as vapes, mods, or e-cigarettes, have become popular over the years. They have tapped into a billion dollar industry, and appear to be staying for good in an ever increasing market. Once touted as a tobacco cessation tool, ENDS have created a sub-niche with many flavors, customizations, and lobbying groups. ENDS, in users eyes, do not hold the stigma associated with combustible tobacco cigarettes. They are perceived as a socially acceptable, healthier alternative that lacks the health detriments of traditional tobacco products. Their target market is not only adults, but also minors, with common flavors such as bubble gum, vanilla, and watermelon. Surveys of young teens have shown that the percentage of minors using ENDS is growing, year over year. The ENDS products themselves also offer different customizations, ranging from longer lasting batteries to larger reservoirs. In regards to regulation, the US Food and

* Corresponding Author's Email: r_pacheco1@u.pacific.edu.

Drug Administration (FDA) recently extended its authority over tobacco products to include ENDS. One such change brought on by the FDA are box labels to warn of nicotine addiction on ENDS products, similar to their combustible counterparts.

Keywords: electronic cigarettes, e-cigs, vapes, pens, pods, tobacco, cessation, advertising, health

COMPOSITION AND STRUCTURE

Types

Electronic nicotine delivery systems (ENDS) work by using a battery (i.e., Li-ion) to atomize an e-liquid into an aerosol/vapor, which the user then inhales and later releases. ENDS are currently available in many forms spanning three generations. Upon the arrival of ENDS in the mid 2000s, the first generation was referred to as cig-a-likes. This form, which was reminiscent of a traditional, combustible cigarette, was instrumental in the early adoption of ENDS in the cigarette cessation market. After some time, the second generation ENDS came to market in the shape of vape/hookah pens, modifications (mods) and reusable electronic cigarettes. Mods opened the customization arena by allowing users to modify their ENDS with refillable reservoirs, varying battery capacities, atomizers, and use e-liquids with nicotine concentrations comparable to combustible cigarettes. Mods allowed individual users to customize their experience for enjoyment. The third generation then arrived, with what are now called pods or pod devices—small electronic units, akin to a USB storage drive. Pods were well received by users as their nicotine delivery speed is similar to that of a combustible cigarette [1, 2].

Looking at market share, first generation ENDS represented 56.9% of dollar sales in 2013. Second and third generation ENDS captured 89.4% of dollar sales by 2017, and increased to 95.3% in 2018 [3]. One explanation for this can be the abundance of flavors offered in second and third generation ENDS. First time ENDS users, who have never previously smoked combustible cigarettes, prefer flavor as it may serve to subdue the taste/feel of nicotine. Users transitioning to ENDS as a form of cessation or substitution, are more likely to pick more traditional tobacco flavors [4].

An example of pod type devices is JUUL, which is a key player in the current market [5]. These pods have allowed adolescent users to go unnoticed by parents as they resemble and blend in with USB storage drives. JUUL devices contain nicotine similar to other ENDS, and because of their style, are more readily accepted as a cigarette alternative [6]. JUULs consist of a rechargeable electronic cigarette, along with replaceable pods. One pod, according to some reports, is comparable to a pack of combustible cigarettes. One article reported that traditional JUUL use ranges from about 4-10 pods per month among occasional-daily users, respectively [7]. In 2016, according to the Centers for Disease Control (CDC), the average combustible cigarette smoker went through 0.7 packs per day, or about 21 packs per month [8]. If we hold the above ratio of 1 pod : 1 pack of cigarettes, it appears that JUUL users in the cessation realm appear to be using less nicotine, and thereby coming closer to quitting tobacco products.

Regulation

When the Family Smoking Prevention and Tobacco Control Act was passed by Congress and signed by President Barack Obama in June 2009, it gave the United States Food and Drug Administration (FDA) full authority to regulate tobacco products, except ENDS. At that time, ENDS were able to enter the market, completely devoid of regulation on the products and advertising. It was not until 2016, when the FDA's authority was finally extended to include ENDS. This extension brought: health warnings on ENDS packages, requirement that ENDS products meet public health standards, and enforcement of the minimum buying age of 18 years old, via photo ID [9].

Under this new extension of authority, ENDS must be approved for marketing by the FDA. The FDA recently extended its deadline for ENDS marketing review applications to August 8, 2022. In other words, for now,

ENDS can still advertise as they were before. After August, 8, 2022, the ENDS product would need to support and protect the public health to receive marketing approval. One example of this would be to show the new product would be used for tobacco cessation among current tobacco users [10].

Brands

The most popular brands keep changing in the ENDS market. As an example, in 2013, the brands that held the largest market share were: blu, NJOY, and Logic. Contrast that to 2017 and 2018, where the new market share leaders were: JUUL, Vuse, and MarkTen [3]. This market is so volatile, that one of these brands, MarkTen, had discontinued all of its products by the end of 2018 [11]. As of 2018, JUUL owned the largest dollar market share at 66.9% [3].

Ingredients

Among the three generations of ENDS, their liquid, or e-liquid, has some commonality. E-liquids can consist of a mixture including nicotine, toxicants (including formaldehyde, diacetyl and acetyl propionyl) and a base (propylene glycol and/or vegetable glycerin) [12-14].

Nicotine concentrations can vary as well. There are some e-liquids that are nicotine free. These are rare, and often confused with e-liquids containing nicotine, often as a result of poor labeling. Nicotine free products generally account for less than 1% of dollar market share. Among first generation e-liquids, the nicotine concentration went as high as 2.7% in 2017. Among second and third generation e-liquids, nicotine concentration went as high as 4.4%. The higher nicotine concentration e-liquids accounted for about 74.7% of dollar market share in 2018 [3]. However, specific concentration of nicotine seems insignificant to users as about a third of past 30-day users, and half of past year users were unsure of the nicotine concentrations of their current e-liquid [15].

JUUL has been dominant in the dollar market share field. This may be a result of the nicotine found in their e-liquid as it is a nicotine salt instead of the more traditional, free-base nicotine. Other ingredients found in JUUL e-liquid are propylene glycol, glycerol, benzoic acid, natural oils, extracts and flavor [5]. Increased levels of free-base nicotine can create a user experience of harshness, with increased irritation to the throat and lungs, also referred to as, "throat hit." Using nicotine salt, with the addition of benzoic acid, the pH can be lowered (made less basic/alkaline), and the harshness and irritability reduced [14, 16, 17].

Nicotine exists in an equilibria of two chemical forms: salt (monoprotonated) and free-base (unprotonated). This equilibria is dependent on the pH of the e-liquid. When the pH is high (basic), more free-base nicotine is available, and when the pH is low (acidic), more salt is present. Nicotine's dissociation constant, or pKa, is 8.02. Therefore, at a pH of 8.02, there exists a perfect equilibria of the two forms. To cross and be absorbed by biological membranes, such as alveoli, the free-base form is needed. Usually e-liquids are buffered to keep an abundance of free-base available, which increases the harshness and irritation. By using benzoic acid, JUUL goes against this norm and therefore, offers a more user friendly experience [16, 18].

Since second and third generation ENDS allow for refill of e-liquids, some users have been able to exploit this and use custom (user-made or store bought) mixtures of e-liquids that contain marijuana, methamphetamine, heroin, and/or methadone. More experienced users of second and third generation ENDS can modify their device to create a bigger, stronger puff with higher drug concentration [14, 19].

Flavors

One of the main reasons for the popularity of ENDS is the abundance of flavors offered by major brands. In fact, one of the main reasons many young adults began using ENDS was the flavors. Amount adults, 43.1% selected fruit as their flavor of choice, followed by mint and menthol at 30.2%, sweet at 29.9%, candy at 24.8% and tobacco at 23.3% [20]. When looking at dollar sales from 2013 to 2017, tobacco and mint/menthol controlled about a third of the market, each. In 2018, fruit increased its dollar sales to 27.7%, while tobacco fell to 14.3%, and mint/menthol was stable at 33.9% [3].

Menthol is a common flavor in ENDS products, as well as traditional tobacco products. One study reported that internal industry files indicate menthol was utilized to help increase appeal [18].

Another ingredient used to increase appeal of flavors is sucrose. In a convenience sample generated with 37 e-liquids from different brands and flavors, sucrose was found in every sample. Concentration ranged from 0.76-72.93 μg/g [18]. This also has an impact on the cariogenicity of e-liquids (See subsection 7.1.1 for more information).

ENDS brands state that their flavors are meant for the enjoyment of the adult crowd, however as much as 81% of adolescents who have ever used an ENDS, recall their first one being flavored [21]. In fact, that first flavored ENDS use often led adolescents to continue usage at 18 months follow up; more-so than those adolescents whose first ENDS was unflavored [22].

ENDS brands have also capitalized on decreased harm perception by using sweet and fruit flavors [23]. Users of flavored e-liquids, such as sweet and fruit, find more satisfaction, and perceived themselves as more addicted to ENDS products, in comparison to users of non-flavored e-liquids. This will aid in justification of the FDA's likely plan to limit e-liquid options to menthol/mint and tobacco [24]. Data has shown that if flavors were more limited, for example, if tobacco was the predominant flavor offered, the entire ENDS line would become less appealing for younger never smokers [4]. In September 2019, President Donald Trump pushed the issue and stated that the FDA would be putting out "some very strong recommendations" in "a couple of weeks." The inference is that after the new guidance is released by the FDA, most, if not all, flavored ENDS will be removed from the market, pending future approval after application [25].

Solution

Nicotine and other ingredients are usually dissolved in a solution of propylene glycol (PG) or vegetable glycerin (VG), and sometimes, a ratio of both. The one difference that has been documented between both liquid solutions, is that PG forms a larger particle size in vapor form, that has been associated with a worsened "throat hit" sensation. As eluded to earlier in subsection 2.4.3, the "throat hit" sensation is experienced during increased irritation or harshness to the throat and lung epithelia [17]. At times, this has been viewed desirably, as users of ENDS attempting to quit or transition over from combustible cigarette use, may want a similar "throat hit." An e-liquid consisting of VG forms a smaller particle size, thereby minimizing the "throat hit" and allowing for a smoother experience [14].

Adolescents

Qualified Adolescent Use

Tobacco use in adolescents has shifted from predominantly combustible cigarettes and smokeless tobacco, towards ENDS. By 2016, ENDS had become the product of choice for tobacco use among high students, according to the National Youth Tobacco Survey [26]. A report put forth by the CDC highlights that about 5% of students in grades 6-8 self reported past 30 day use of an ENDS product [27, 28]. In grades 9-12, self reported past 30 day use increased to 20.8% [27]. Among high school students who report ever using ENDS, about 64% reference use of a JUUL product, sometimes in conjunction with other ENDS. About 47% of current use high school students report using JUUL [2]. Furthermore, in regards to first use of nicotine-free or nicotine containing ENDS products, there was a strong association with continued use during first year of high school for nicotine containing ENDS among students [22].

Motivators for Adolescent Use

As previously discussed in section 2.5, flavors have had a big role in attracting young adult previous smokers, and never smokers. Flavors have also had an impact on attracting adolescents to first time use. Other common reasons cited by adolescents for ENDS usage were: coolness factor, easy to hide, cheaper, peer influences, lack of the traditional tobacco smell, and futuristic [21, 29, 30]. In regards to peer influences, adolescents were more likely to report having immediate family and close friends who had used ENDS and combustible cigarettes [29]. Data also reveals that among never smoking adolescents, those with elevated use of electronic devices were more likely to try ENDS when older [31]. Since adolescent use of an ENDS product is a strong predictor for use of other tobacco products, accessibility is also an area now being more closely monitored [2]. The FDA recently (September 2018) issued over 1,300 penalty fines and warning letters to retailers who had previously sold ENDS to adolescents under the age of 18 [32].

Naive Adolescents

Another concerning issue with adolescent ENDS use is their lack of knowledge of the product which they are using. When asked about the vapor produced by ENDS, about 19% of adolescents reported it was water. About 23% of adolescents did not consider ENDS as tobacco products, and about 43% felt ENDS were safer than using a combustible cigarette [29]. In addition, many past 30 day use adolescents were unable to recall if the ENDS they had used contained any nicotine [2].

Parental Views

Parents of adolescents are aware of the dangers ENDS pose for their children, but many are not educated on the current products or their subsequent use. In a recent survey of parents, about 55% were able to recall JUUL as a brand of ENDS, yet about only 44% were able to accurately identify a JUUL product. Many parents were concerned about ENDS usage among adolescents, but only about 32% reported concern of use among their own children [33]. Considering adolescent ENDS use has the potential to have long lasting effects on the brain's behavior and development, possibly increasing susceptibility to future drug abuse, parents need to be more protective of their children, and not wait for information to be disseminated to them intrinsically [34-36].

ADVERTISING

Marketing

For the last few decades, combustible cigarette and tobacco advertising has been banned from TV and radio [28]. As previously discussed in section 2.3, the FDA recently had their authority extended and by 2022, all ENDS marketing will need FDA approval prior to release. As a result, ENDS marketing has gone unregulated, and expenditures have been on the rise. In 2011, ENDS brands spent $6.4 million on marketing. In 2012, just one year later, that number nearly tripled to $18.3 million, with the largest amounts being spent on magazine and television ads by over 80 brands [37].

Youth Exposure

ENDS brands will deny advertising directed towards youth, however, their marketing strategies tell a different truth. Between 2011 and 2013, adolescent exposure to television ads for ENDS increased about 256% [38]. By 2016, ENDS advertisements in retailers had become the most common source for ENDS exposure to adolescents, followed closely by television, internet and social media [39-41]. Adolescents are cognizant of ENDS advertisements. More than ⅓ of youth who recalled seeing an ENDS advertisement in the previous month had found them to be appealing [40]. In 2015, about 38% of youth surveyed did recall seeing ENDS advertisements. This survey demonstrated these youth with exposure to ENDS advertising were at increased odds to use ENDS [41]. A growing number of ENDS advertisements have also been seen on the social media platform Facebook. These advertisements target at youth, were strongly associated with conversion of non-smokers into ENDS users in youth viewers [42]. Advertisements are designed to appeal to a product's audience. For example, non-white female youth, with a history of previous cigarette smoking or ENDS use, were more likely to find ENDS advertisements appealing, in comparison to youth with no history of use [40]. In another example, repeated exposure to ENDS advertisements online and in retailers can double the odds of a current never-smoker adolescent to start use upon early adulthood [43].

CESSATION

Vehicle for Cessation

Upon market entry, ENDS were touted as a route for tobacco cessation. There is some truth to the above statement. For example, in one study using ENDS as a tobacco cessation tool in comparison to nicotine replacement therapy (NRT), 3 people were able to quit successfully using ENDS for every 1 person who quit using NRT [44]. ENDS have been endorsed by Public Health England for tobacco cessation [40]. ENDS are an alternative to combustible cigarettes. In some considerations, they are less harmful, and have been shown improve a smoker's health [45].

Gateway to Addiction

When used as a tobacco cessation tool, ENDS can find purpose. However, they have also been able to convert never-smokers into current users. Among a group of adolescents surveyed, use of ENDS was "positively and independently" shown to lead towards use of combustible cigarettes [46]. Another survey also found that youth were more likely to use ENDS as a way to bypass smoking restrictions, not aimed cessation [47].

EXPLOSIONS

Dental

ENDS explosions can cause severe harm to the dentition and oral cavity. In one case study, an explosion and subsequent fire occurred during use of a relatively new ENDS (11 days of use), resulting in luxation (movement) of teeth, avulsion (loss) of teeth, and fractures to maxillary bones and burns to epithelia [48].

Burns

Burns associated with explosions and fires have been so common, that after a series of case studies, one group pioneered the following classification system for burns: Type A: thermal burn in conjunction with flames as a result of the internal battery overheating to combustion; Type B: burn secondary to the explosion itself; Type C: chemical burn from the battery's solution; and Type D: thermal burn from improper use [49]. Burn patients were most commonly male, and the front pocket area on the legs were the most common burn site [50]. Hospitals are beginning to see and become more accustomed to treating these burn patients. For example, during a 6 month period from 2015-2016, the Santa Clara Valley Medical Center Burn Unit treated three severe burn patients as a result of combustion of an ENDS, two of which were hospitalized [51]. In another series of case studies analyzing 47 burn patients as a result of combusting/exploding ENDS, fractures were recorded on two cervical vertebra and one palate, three teeth appeared damaged, and 37 thermal/chemical burns [52].

HEALTH

Dental

When ENDS users inhale, one of the first systems to come into contact with the vapor is the oral cavity. ENDS users have increased odds of developing periodontal disease and incurring alveolar bone loss around teeth, causing teeth to become more mobile. These odds increased with subsequent marijuana use and illicit drug use [53]. ENDS vapor has been shown to quadruple microbial adhesion to enamel, in formation of a stronger biofilm. If the vapor was flavored, biofilm formation doubled and a subsequent decrease of 27% was detected in enamel hardness (in comparison to unflavored vapor). The viscosity of the vapor supports *Streptococcus mutans* adhesion to dental enamel [54]. *S. mutans* is a cariogenic bacteria present in the oral cavity responsible for creating carious lesions. *S. mutans* acts by breaking down sucrose (subsection 2.5.3) to form lactic acid, which weakens enamel via demineralization. If this process proceeds for a long time, a carious lesion (cavity) will form that will require attention by a dentist.

Pulmonary

After the mouth, the next system to endure the vapor is the respiratory system. ENDS have been associated with respiratory symptoms in adolescents, such as asthma, airway inflammation, airway resistance, chronic bronchitis, and pulmonary toxicity [55-58]. Exposure to ENDS vapor has been shown in lab studies to be cytotoxic to airway cells, as well as diminish antimicrobial properties of macrophages and neutrophils [59]. One study found that a majority of e-liquids contained diacetyl and acetyl propionyl. Diacetyl is known for its role in causing bronchiolitis obliterans [12, 60].

Cardiovascular

Lastly, within the pulmonary system, the vapor finally comes into contact with alveoli and can transfer the blood-air barrier (alveolar-capillary membrane). ENDS have been shown to increase heart rate and diastolic blood pressure [45]. Even nicotine free e-liquids have been shown to affect endothelial function [61].

Carcinogens

Carcinogens were detectable in adolescent urine excretions of ENDS only users. These included metabolites of "acrylonitrile, acrolein, propylene oxide, acrylamide, and crotonaldehyde" [62]. The presence of the above metabolites of carcinogens in urine disproves any claim ENDS brands may attempt to make in relation to safety and healthier aspects of their products. In another study, the carcinogenic metals "cadmium, chromium, lead, manganese and nickel" were present in common e-liquids used [63].

Morbidity

In total, 18 people in the United States have died after developing a lung disease subsequent to use of ENDS. As of October 1, 2019, the CDC has been informed of 1,080 patients with similar lung symptoms across the US; a majority of whom report previous use an ENDS containing tetrahydrocannabinol (THC) [64].

Adult Use

Qualified Adult Use

Adult use of ENDS ranges from recreational/social to cessation. In one survey of current adult ENDS users, 51.4% were trying out ENDS and

81.7% had past 30 day history of combustible cigarette use. This study also observed that adult ENDS users were more likely to be "younger, white males with lower education and income" [30]. The above survey statistics supports the cessation aspect of ENDS use. In addition, other reasons for ENDS use includes the abundance of flavors, the variety of new products available, cigarette alternatives, nicer smell and healthier when compared to combustible cigarettes, and peer influence from friends [20, 30].

Marijuana Co-Use

Studies show that some ENDS users are also likely to use marijuana. One study in particular stated that ENDS users were 2.5-4 times more likely to use marijuana products as well [19]. Another correlation seen was ENDS use at the age of 14 increased the likelihood of beginning to use marijuana about 2 years later [65].

Conclusion

Electronic nicotine delivery systems originally came to market with aspirations of an amazing tobacco cessation tool for individuals who had previously struggled to quit. Fast forward some years, and the market has developed and changed drastically. ENDS adolescent use is now recorded as early as 6th grade, and adolescent progression to combustible cigarette use has been documented as well. With more users, health implications are starting to come to realization, as well as accidental physical injuries from use. The impending FDA regulations only show that the ENDS market will continue to evolve and adapt.

REFERENCES

[1] Wagener, T.L., et al., Have combustible cigarettes met their match? The nicotine delivery profiles and harmful constituent exposures of second-generation and third-generation electronic cigarette users. *Tob Control,* 2017. 26(e1): p. e23-e28.

[2] Krishnan-Sarin, S., et al., E-cigarette devices used by high-school youth. *Drug Alcohol Depend*, 2019. 194: p. 395-400.

[3] Romberg, A. R., et al., Patterns of nicotine concentrations in electronic cigarettes sold in the United States, 2013-2018. *Drug Alcohol Depend*, 2019. 203: p. 1-7.

[4] Leventhal, A. M., et al., Effects of non-tobacco flavors and nicotine on e-cigarette product appeal among young adult never, former, and current smokers. *Drug Alcohol Depend*, 2019. 203: p. 99-106.

[5] Fadus, M. C., T.T. Smith, and L.M. Squeglia, The rise of e-cigarettes, pod mod devices, and JUUL among youth: Factors influencing use, health implications, and downstream effects. *Drug Alcohol Depend,* 2019. 201: p. 85-93.

[6] Nardone, N., et al., JUUL electronic cigarettes: Nicotine exposure and the user experience. *Drug Alcohol Depend,* 2019. 203: p. 83-87.

[7] Leavens, E. L. S., et al., JUUL electronic cigarette use patterns, other tobacco product use, and reasons for use among ever users: Results from a convenience sample. *Addict Behav*, 2019. 95: p. 178-183.

[8] CDC. *Smoking is down, but almost 38 million American adults still smoke*. 2018 [cited 2019 October 10]; Available from: https://www.cdc.gov/media/releases/2018/p0118-smoking-rates-declining.html.

[9] USFDA. *The Facts on the FDA's New Tobacco Rule*. 2016 [cited 2019 10/3/2019]; Available from: https://www.fda.gov/consumers/consumer-updates/facts-fdas-new-tobacco-rule.

[10] *Truth E-Cigarette Fact Sheet*. 2018 October 3, 2019]; Available from: https://truthinitiative.org/sites/default/files/media/files/2019/03/Truth_E-Cigarette_FactSheet_FINAL.pdf.

[11] MarkTen. *MarkTen® Discontinuation Announcement.* 2018 10/4/2019]; Available from: http://www.markten.com.

[12] Farsalinos, K. E., et al., Evaluation of electronic cigarette liquids and aerosol for the presence of selected inhalation toxins. *Nicotine Tob Res,* 2015. 17(2): p. 168-174.

[13] Logue, J. M., et al., Emissions from Electronic Cigarettes: Assessing Vapers' Intake of Toxic Compounds, Secondhand Exposures, and the Associated Health Impacts. *Environmental Science & Technology,* 2017. 51(16): p. 9271-9279.

[14] Mulder, H. A., et al., The Effect of Electronic Cigarette User Modifications and E-liquid Adulteration on the Particle Size Profile of an Aerosolized Product. *Sci Rep,* 2019. 9(1): p. 10221.

[15] Parker, M. A., J. L. Pearson, and A. C. Villanti, Limited utility of detailed e-cigarette use measures: An analysis of NESARC-III. *Addict Behav,* 2019. 97: p. 56-62.

[16] Duell, A. K., J. F. Pankow, and D. H. Peyton, Free-Base Nicotine Determination in Electronic Cigarette Liquids by (1)H NMR Spectroscopy. *Chem Res Toxicol*, 2018. 31(6): p. 431-434.

[17] *PG vs VG Eliquid and how it affects Vaping performance*. Veppo Vape Shop 2019; Available from: https://veppocig.com/pg-vs-vg-eliquid/.

[18] DeVito, E. E. and S. Krishnan-Sarin, E-cigarettes: Impact of E-Liquid Components and Device Characteristics on Nicotine Exposure. *Curr Neuropharmacol,* 2018. 16(4): p. 438-459.

[19] Nguyen, N., et al., Past 30-day co-use of tobacco and marijuana products among adolescents and young adults in California. *Addict Behav,* 2019. 98: p. 106053.

[20] Vu, T. T., et al., Age differences in electronic nicotine delivery systems (ENDS) usage motivations and behaviors, perceived health benefit, and intention to quit. *Addict Behav*, 2019. 98: p. 106054.

[21] Ambrose, B. K., et al., Flavored Tobacco Product Use Among US Youth Aged 12-17 Years, 2013-2014. *JAMA*, 2015. 314(17): p. 1871-1873.

[22] Audrain-McGovern, J., et al., Initial e-cigarette flavoring and nicotine exposure and e-cigarette uptake among adolescents. *Drug Alcohol Depend,* 2019. 202: p. 149-155.

[23] Zare, S., M. Nemati, and Y. Zheng, A systematic review of consumer preference for e-cigarette attributes: Flavor, nicotine strength, and type. *PLoS One*, 2018. 13(3): p. e0194145.

[24] Landry, R. L., et al., The role of flavors in vaping initiation and satisfaction among U.S. adults. *Addict Behav*, 2019. 99: p. 106077.

[25] Vazquez, M. and B. Klein. *Trump administration moves to ban flavored e-cigarettes*. Politics 2019 September 11, 2019 [cited 2019 10/4/2019]; Available from: https://www.cnn.com/2019/09/11/politics/donald-trump-vape-e-cigarette-flavors/index.html.

[26] Jamal, A., et al., Tobacco Use Among Middle and High School Students — United States, 2011–2016. *Morbidity and Mortality Weekly Report,* 2017. 66(23): p. 597-603.

[27] Cullen, K. A., et al., Tobacco Product Use Among Middle and High School Students - United States, 2011-2017. *MMWR Morb Mortal Wkly Rep,* 2018. 67(45): p. 1276-1277.

[28] Andrews, M. *Juul And Other E-Cig Makers Are Free To Advertise, Though Big Tobacco Can't.* Shots 2019 August 20, 2019 October 3, 2019]; August 20, 2019:[Available from: https://www.npr.org/sections/health-shots/2019/08/20/752553108/cigarettes-cant-be-advertised-on-tv-should-juul-ads-be-permitted.

[29] Gorukanti, A., et al., Adolescents' attitudes towards e-cigarette ingredients, safety, addictive properties, social norms, and regulation. *Prev Med,* 2017. 94: p. 65-71.

[30] Nicksic, N. E., L.M. Snell, and A.J. Barnes, Reasons to use e-cigarettes among adults and youth in the Population Assessment of Tobacco and Health (PATH) study. *Addict Behav*, 2019. 93: p. 93-99.

[31] Lee, S., et al., A prospective longitudinal relation between elevated use of electronic devices and use of electronic nicotine delivery systems. *Addict Behav*, 2019. 98: p. 106063.

[32] US Department of Health and Human Services, F.a.D.A., FDA takes new steps to address epidemic of youth e-cigarette use, including a

historic action against more than 1,300 retailers and 5 major manufacturers for their roles perpetuating youth access [press release], F.a.D.A. US Department of Health and Human Services, Editor. 2018, US Department of Health and Human Services, *Food and Drug Administration;*.

[33] Patel, M., et al., Parents' Awareness and Perceptions of JUUL and Other E-Cigarettes. *Am J Prev Med,* 2019.

[34] Yuan, M., et al., Nicotine and the adolescent brain. *J Physiol*, 2015. 593(16): p. 3397-3412.

[35] Squeglia, L. M. and K. M. Gray, Alcohol and Drug Use and the Developing Brain. *Current Psychiatry Reports,* 2016. 18(46).

[36] Ren, M. and S. Lotfipour, Nicotine gateway effects on adolescent substance use. *Western Journal of Emergency Medicine*, 2019. 20(5): p. 696-709.

[37] Kim, A. E., K. Y. Arnold, and O. Makarenko, E-cigarette advertising expenditures in the U.S., 2011-2012. *Am J Prev Med,* 2014. 46(4): p. 409-412.

[38] *Vaporized Youth Exposure To E-Cigarette Marketing*. 2015; Available from: https://truthinitiative.org/sites/default/files/media/files/2019/03/Vaporized-Youth-Exposure-To-E-Cigarette-Marketing.pdf.

[39] Marynak, K., et al., Exposure to electronic cigarette advertising among middle and high school students — United Utates, 2014–2016. Morbidity and Mortality *Weekly Report,* 2018. 67(10): p. 294-299.

[40] Cho, Y. J., et al., Youth self-reported exposure to and perceptions of vaping advertisements: Findings from the 2017 International Tobacco Control Youth Tobacco and Vaping Survey. *Prev Med*, 2019. 126: p. 105775.

[41] Papaleontiou, L., I. T. Agaku, and F. T. Filippidis, Effects of Exposure to Tobacco and Electronic Cigarette Advertisements on Tobacco Use: An Analysis of the 2015 National Youth Tobacco Survey. *J Adolesc Health,* 2019.

[42] Camenga, D., et al., E-cigarette advertising exposure in e-cigarette naive adolescents and subsequent e-cigarette use: A longitudinal cohort study. *Addict Behav*, 2018. 81: p. 78-83.

[43] Cruz, T. B., et al., Tobacco Marketing and Subsequent Use of Cigarettes, E-Cigarettes, and Hookah in Adolescents. *Nicotine Tob Res,* 2019. 21(7): p. 926-932.

[44] Cox, S., et al., Effects of e-cigarettes versus nicotine replacement therapy on short-term smoking abstinence when delivered at a community pharmacy. *Addict Behav Rep*, 2019. 10: p. 100202.

[45] Yan, X. S. and C. D'Ruiz, Effects of using electronic cigarettes on nicotine delivery and cardiovascular function in comparison with regular cigarettes. *Regul Toxicol Pharmacol*, 2015. 71(1): p. 24-34.

[46] Chaffee, B. W., S. L. Watkins, and S. A. Glantz, Electronic Cigarette Use and Progression From Experimentation to Established Smoking. *Pediatrics,* 2018. 141(4).

[47] Tucker, J. S., et al., Alternative tobacco product use and smoking cessation among homeless youth in los angeles county. *Nicotine Tob Res*, 2014. 16(11): p. 1522-6.

[48] Harrison, R. and D. Hicklin, Jr., Electronic cigarette explosions involving the oral cavity. *J Am Dent Assoc,* 2016. 147(11): p. 891-896.

[49] Serror, K., et al., Burns caused by electronic vaping devices (e-cigarettes): A new classification proposal based on mechanisms. *Burns,* 2018. 44(3): p. 544-548.

[50] Hickey, S., et al., Thermal injuries from exploding electronic cigarettes. *Burns,* 2018. 44(5): p. 1294-1301.

[51] Sheckter, C., et al., Burns resulting from spontaneous combustion of electronic cigarettes: a case series. *Burns Trauma,* 2016. 4: p. 35.

[52] Rudy, S. F. and E.L. Durmowicz, Electronic nicotine delivery systems: overheating, fires and explosions. *Tob Control*, 2016. 26: p. 10-18.

[53] Atuegwu, N. C., et al., Association between Regular Electronic Nicotine Product Use and Self-reported Periodontal Disease Status: Population Assessment of Tobacco and Health Survey. *Int J Environ Res Public Health*, 2019. 16(7).

[54] Kim, S. A., et al., Cariogenic potential of sweet flavors in electronic-cigarette liquids. *PLoS One*, 2018. 13(9): p. e0203717.

[55] Cho, J. H. and S.Y. Paik, Association between Electronic Cigarette Use and Asthma among High School Students in South Korea. *PLoS One,* 2016. 11(3): p. 1-13.

[56] Wang, M. P., et al., Electronic Cigarette Use and Respiratory Symptoms in Chinese Adolescents in Hong Kong. *JAMA Pediatrics*, 2016. 170(1): p. 89-91.

[57] Chun, L. F., et al., Pulmonary toxicity of e-cigarettes. *Am J Physiol Lung Cell Mol Physiol,* 2017. 313(2): p. L193-L206.

[58] McConnell, R., et al., Electronic Cigarette Use and Respiratory Symptoms in Adolescents. *Am J Respir Crit Care Med,* 2017. 195(8): p. 1043-1049.

[59] Hwang, J. H., et al., Electronic cigarette inhalation alters innate immunity and airway cytokines while increasing the virulence of colonizing bacteria. *Journal of Molecular Medicine*, 2016. 94(6): p. 667–679.

[60] Park, R. and S. Gilbert, Pulmonary Impairment and Risk Assessment in a Diacetyl-Exposed Population: Microwave Popcorn Workers. *J Occup Environ Med*, 2018. 60(6): p. 496-506.

[61] Caporale, A., et al., Acute Effects of Electronic Cigarette Aerosol Inhalation on Vascular Function Detected at Quantitative MRI. *Radiology*, 2019. 293(1): p. 97-106.

[62] Rubinstein, M. L., et al., Adolescent Exposure to Toxic Volatile Organic Chemicals From E-Cigarettes. *Pediatrics,* 2018. 141(4).

[63] Hess, C. A., et al., E-cigarettes as a source of toxic and potentially carcinogenic metals. *Environ Res,* 2017. 152: p. 221-225.

[64] CDC. *Outbreak of Lung Injury Associated with E-Cigarette Use, or Vaping*. 2019 [cited 2019 October 8, 2019]; Available from: https://www.cdc.gov/tobacco/basic_information/e-cigarettes/severe-lung-disease.html.

[65] Audrain-McGovern, J., et al., Adolescent E-Cigarette, Hookah, and Conventional Cigarette Use and Subsequent Marijuana Use. *Pediatrics*, 2018. 142(3).

In: New Research on Tobacco
Editor: Uta Dreher
ISBN: 978-1-53617-077-1

Chapter 4

AGE OF INITIATION OF TOBACCO CONSUMPTION IN INDIA: EVIDENCE FROM GLOBAL ADULT TOBACCO SURVEY DATA

***Jitendra Gupta*[1], *Ramu Rawat*[1,*]**
***and Afsaneh Mirzaei*[2]**
[1]Department of Mathematical Demography and Statistics,
IIPS, Mumbai, India
[2]Islamic Azad University, Tehran, Iran

ABSTRACT

This study examines the early and late age at initiation of tobacco consumption in India. It uses Global Adult Tobacco Survey (2009-10) data to this end. Bivariate and multivariate statistical techniques are used to analyze the data set. The findings reveal that the respondents living in rural areas were highly initiated in different forms of tobacco as compared with urban space. Education was one of the primary factors for initiation of

---

* Corresponding Author's Email: ramu.iips@gmail.com.

tobacco use. Respondents having secondary and above education were highly initiated in late age. However, the age of tobacco initiation either early or late was significantly higher (7 per cent) among males as compared with females. Respondents belonging to the central (4.9 per cent) and northern regions (4.6 per cent) were highly initiated to tobacco as compared with other regions. Considering a decline in the initiation of tobacco consumption, local level awareness and catchy programmes play an effective role. In this, the involvement of children, women and leaders can be help to reach the goal.

Keywords: smoking tobacco, smokeless tobacco, consumption and initiation

INTRODUCTION

According to WHO's estimate, one person dies every six seconds due to tobacco consumption, which accounts for one in 10 adult deaths, while more than half of current users will eventually die of a tobacco-related disease. Globally, about 10 million people will die by 2030 because of high tobacco consumption and 70 per cent deaths occur in developing countries. Tobacco consumption rate in different forms is estimated to be higher in developing countries. India is the second largest country in the world as a tobacco producer and consumer. It accounts for about 10 per cent of the world's tobacco cultivated area (about 4 million hectares) and 9 per cent of global production with about 1.3 billion people engaged in tobacco production. While about 9 million people die each year in India due to tobacco use. Among them, 30 percent deaths are by cancer with 7 per cent death occurring among people aged 30 years and above. Taking into consideration all this, India plays a key role at the global level to control tobacco consumption and to warn the people about the serious health hazards caused by it. There are more tobacco-related deaths here than from any other cause and more than the combined deaths from pneumonia, diarrheal diseases, tuberculosis and complications of childbirth (Jha and Chaloupka 2000; Jha et al. 2002). Although tobacco consumption has increased across the world, its high use has been reported in developing countries. Smoking tobacco increased dramatically among children and adults where it accounts from 4.9 per cent to 14.3 per cent and 4.9 per cent to 14.3 per cent respectively. For smokeless tobacco the figures varied from 1.2 per cent to 10.2 per cent and 1.3 per cent to 8.7 per cent for middle school and high school children before 11 years of age respectively (Gupta and Ray 2002 and 2007; Jha and Chaloupka 2000; CDC 1998).

Tobacco consumption is a pediatric epidemic around the world. It increased from 49 to 61 per cent from 1976 to 2000 in developing countries. The latter are expected to account for about 71 per cent of global tobacco consumption (Mackay et al. 1996). Nearly 29 per cent, i.e., 1.1 billion of the world's adult population, smoked daily (Jha and Chaloupka 2000; CDC 1998). According to Doll et al. 2004, approximately 80 per cent population begins tobacco consumption during childhood and half of it dies 13 years earlier as compared to his or her peers who are non-tobacco users. Furthermore, the previous study documented that two out of three 12th graders who were current smokers had started smoking by the end of the ninth grade, and at the end of high school, 43.6 per cent of all kids tried smoking (Johnston et al. 2010). One study was done on high school students in United Nation or Kingdom? It shows that the about 14 per cent students had smoked at least one entire cigarette before the age of 13 years, with more ninth-graders (16.3 per cent) having smoked a full cigarette than 12th graders (13.3 per cent) (Eaton et al. 2010). Therefore, the critical finding was that more than a third of all kids who ever try smoking a cigarette become regular and daily smokers before leaving high school. Tobacco consumption became an addiction for young people and, therefore, cessation of its consumption was problematic and early quitting may be difficult (Riggs et al. 2007). The one study shows that a majority of young people increasingly think of tobacco consumption in working hours, while obese people thought that the use of tobacco helped to reduce body weight (Bean et al. 2008). However, a higher percentage of people use smokeless tobacco? during childhood, whereas later they start tobacco consumption. Furthermore, the high use of any form of tobacco consumption increases the probability of morbidity, especial mouth cancer and other diseases, and sometimes morbidity may end in death (Morris et al. 2011; Eaton et al. 2010).

A study conducted in Nairobi (2004) shows that nearly 72 per cent students were initiated to tobacco in the age group of 12-16 years, whereas, two in every five daily tobacco users aged 20-34 years had started using tobacco daily before attaining? (Kwamanga et al. 2004). According to the Archives of Paediatric and Adolescent Medicine (2007), some youths experience tobacco dependence within a day of first inhaling among their peers (DiFranza et al. 2007). People starting tobacco consumption from childhood have higher health risks like mouth/lung cancer or experience a range of risk factors during adulthood/old age (Dikshit and Kanhere 2000; Hegmann et al. 1993). There was also evidence that smoking was sometimes the first step towards other substance abuse. Therefore, stopping or delaying that first step will reduce the risk that kids will face subsequently (Chaloupka et al. 1999). In India, the use of tobacco has a wide scope because a vast spectrum of tobacco products are easily available for smoking as well as smokeless uses and are relatively cheap (Gupta 2006). Little research has been done on the prevalence and initiation of smoking and smokeless tobacco use. It is well-known that tobacco initiation is a key that determines the future health consequences for the whole society (Kumar et al. 2006; Bhojani et al. 2006; Merrill et al. 1994; Singh and Ladusingh 2014).

According to Sinha's estimation, the risks of tobacco consumption are higher among those who start early and continue its use for an extended period (Morris et al. 2011; Sinha 2002). The most common reasons cited for the children to start using tobacco products are peer pressure, pocket money, easy availability and family member's tobacco consumption habits (Mohan 2005). The initiation and prevalence of tobacco consumption increased from two to four times among the school children according to their grade (VIth – VIIIth) (Reddy et al. 2005). Furthermore, lifetime smoking and other tobacco products consumption usually begins with childhood and high school. Nearly one in 10 in adolescent age group of 13-15 years has ever smoked cigarettes and almost half of the reports say tobacco use started before 10 years of age in India (Sinha et al. 2006). The data presented in the NFHS-3 on current smokers in India from different age groups and by sex demonstrated the prevalence of smoking to be 23? among people aged 30 years and above (IIPS 2007). In the rural areas of Gujarat, Tamil Nadu, Karnataka and Goa one-third to one-half of the children under the age group 10 years experimented with smoking or smokeless tobacco in some form or the other (Pednekar and Gupta 2004; Krishnamurthy et al. 1997). The early age of initiation of tobacco consumption underscores the urgent need to intervene and protect this vulnerable group from falling to addiction (Reddy et al. 2005; Reddy et al. 2004). In this context, the study assessed the prevalence of early and late age initiation of tobacco consumption in India by different selected background characteristics.

Data and Methods

The Global Adult Tobacco Survey (GATS) India that was conducted during 2009-10 have been used for the study. It was conducted in India as a household survey of persons aged 15 years and above by International Institute for Population Sciences, Mumbai. The Survey is the global standard for systematically monitoring adult tobacco use (smoking and smokeless) and tracking key tobacco control indicators. It is a nationally representative household survey designed to produce internationally comparable data on tobacco use and tobacco control indicators using a standardized questionnaire, sampling design, data collection and management procedures. It used multistage sampling procedures. In urban areas three-stage sampling was adopted for the selection of households. About 69,296 respondents were selected among which 33,767 were males and 35,529 females. Out of all the completed interviews, 41,825 were conducted in the rural areas and 27,471 in urban areas. In the GATS survey, India was divided into six regions, viz. northern, central, eastern, western, southern and northeast. The target population for the survey is defined as all Indian residents, aged 15 years and above, and living in their primary residence before the survey date.

Variables under Study

In the study, two sets of variables were included such as response and predictors variables. The following variables were:

Response Variables

Age at initiation of smoking tobacco consumption: This information was collected for a wide variety of smoking tobacco, *i.e.,* cigarettes, cigars, *chillum, chhutta, hookah, chillum (local name)*, etc., products. Age of smoking tobacco products use is categorized as early age and late age in this study. All types of smoking tobacco products are computed as a dichotomous variable (yes '1', no '0').

Age at initiation of smokeless tobacco consumption: The information was collected on items like gutkha, khaini, paan masala, hookah, gul, mawa, misri, etc. Use of these items by the individual has been categorized as early age and late age in this study. Furthermore, all types of smokeless tobacco products are computed as a dichotomous variable (yes '1', no '0').

Predictor Variables

This section includes variables which were affected by the response variable. The determinants are selected based on existing literature and data availability. The determinants involved in the study were the type of residence, sex, age, educational level, occupation, etc.

DATA ANALYTIC STRATEGY

The data was treated with bivariate, multivariate and binary logistic regression statistical techniques to test the significance of analysis by selected indicators on early and late age at initiation of tobacco. The age at initiation of smoking and smokeless tobacco were defined by taking ages below 18 years as early age and 18-24 years as of late age. The binary logistic regression model is commonly estimated by the maximum likelihood function (Retherford and Choe 1993). For each of those outcomes mentioned above variables, the logistic model takes the following general form:

$$\text{Logit } P = \text{Ln } [p/(1-p)] = b_0 + b_1 x_1 + b_2 x_2 + \ldots\ldots + b_i x_i + e_i$$

where, b_1, b_2,.........b_i represents the coefficient of each of the predictor variables included in the model. While e_i is an error term. Ln (P/1-P) represents the natural logarithm of the odds outcome.

RESULTS

Table 1 presents the prevalence and differential of early and late age at initiation of smoking tobacco by different background characteristics in India. In the country, 4 per cent of respondents started smoking tobacco at an early age, while 6.3 per cent respondents began at a late age. There are sex differentials by the initiation of smoking tobacco. However, a higher prevalence of early smoking tobacco has been found among males in early and late ages (7 per cent and 10.8 per cent respectively) as compared with females (0.8 per cent and 1.5 per cent respectively). Respondents from the age group of 55-64 years have initiated smoking tobacco in early age (5.8 per cent) and late age (12.4 per cent) that is higher than other age groups; while in the age group of 15-24 years are significantly less by smoking tobacco (Neufeld et al. 2005) which is also evident in the present study. In the rural area, about 4.4 per cent respondents have initiated tobacco consumption at an early age although in the urban area it is only 2.9 per cent. Late age of initiation of smoking tobacco is significantly higher in the rural area as compared with their urban counterpart. Respondents without formal education and less than primary education have higher initiation of smoking tobacco in the early age group as compared with other educational groups (5.1 per cent and 6.9 per cent respectively) which is corroborated by the study carried out by Sinha et al. (2012).

Table 1. Prevalence of early and late age at initiation of smoking tobacco consumption by selected background characteristics in India, 2009-10

Background characteristics	Age at initiation of smoking tobacco consumption			
	Early		Late	
	%	N	%	N
Place of residence				
Rural	4.4	2319	6.7	3369
Urban	2.9	1023	5.2	1696
Sex				
Male	7.0	3062	10.8	4453
Female	0.8	280	1.5	612
Age group (years)				
15-24	1.9	407	0.7	116
25-44	4.4	1727	6.4	2438
45-54	5.4	581	12.3	1258
55-64	5.8	335	12.4	702
65 and above	5.6	292	10.8	551
Education level				
No formal schooling	5.1	1085	8.3	1677
Less than primary	6.9	582	8.7	785
Primary but less than secondary	3.6	1049	5.2	1332
Secondary and above	2.7	6026	4.0	1271
Occupation				
Govt. & non-Govt. employed	5.7	972	9.7	1698
Self-employed	6.7	1762	9.9	2367
Student	0.6	89	0.2	26
Homemaker	1.1	260	1.8	508
Retired and unemployed	5.3	251	9.5	466
National region				
North	4.6	775	6.8	1294
Central	4.9	544	7.0	756
East	3.8	342	6.2	599
North-east	4.8	1062	7.2	1297
West	2.5	218	3.8	365
South	3.5	401	6.6	754
India	4.0	3342	6.3	5065

Table 2. Logistic regression analysis of early and late age at initiation of smoking tobacco consumption by selected background characteristics in India, 2009-10

Background characteristics	Age at initiation of smoking tobacco consumption	
	Early	Late
	ORs(L-U)	ORs(L-U)
Place of residence		
Rural®		
Urban	0.97 (0.89-1.05)	0.92**(0.86-0.99)
Sex		
Male®		
Female	0.07***(0.06-0.09)	0.12***(0.11-0.13)
Age (years)		
15-24®		
25-44	1.13*(1.00-1.28)	5.73***(4.70-6.99)
45-54	1.07 (0.92-1.23)	9.63***(7.85-11.82)
55-64	1.11 (0.94-1.31)	9.60***(7.76-11.87)
65 and above	1.14 (0.96-1.36)	8.82***(7.08-10.99)
Education level		
No formal schooling®		
Less than primary	0.86***(0.77-0.97)	0.86***(0.78-0.95)
Primary but less than secondary	0.60***(0.55-0.66)	0.63***(0.58-0.68)
Secondary and above	0.27***(0.24-0.30)	0.46***(0.42-0.50)
Occupation		
Govt. & non Govt. employed®		
Self-employed	1.07 (0.98-1.18)	0.90***(0.84-0.97)
Student	0.42***(0.33-0.53)	0.23***(0.15-0.35)
Homemaker	0.82**(0.68-0.98)	0.69***(0.60-0.79)
Retired and unemployed	0.77***(0.66-0.90)	0.76***(0.67-0.86)
National Region		
North®		
Central	0.75***(0.67-0.85)	0.67***(0.61-0.74)
East	0.50***(0.44-0.57)	0.53***(0.47-0.59)
North-east	1.14**(1.03-1.26)	0.83***(0.76-0.91)
West	0.36***(0.31-0.42)	0.34***(0.30-0.39)
South	0.55***(0.49-0.63)	0.59***(0.54-0.65)

Note: ®Reference category; statistically significant at $*p < 0.10$, $**p < 0.05$, $***p < 0.01$.

However, respondents without formal education and less than primary education were initiated in smoking tobacco in the late age were more than those initiated in the respective groups (8.3 percent and 8.7 per cent respectively). Self-employed respondents have higher initiation of smoking tobacco in both early age (6.7 per cent) and late age (9.9 per cent) vis-a-vis their respective counterpart. Persons in the central and north-east regions were more initiated with smoking tobacco than other regions in both early and late ages than their respective counterparts. Western region has the lowest initiation of smoking tobacco than their counterparts WHERE? of both early age (2.5 per cent) and late age (3.8 per cent).Table 2 explains the results of the logistic regression of smoking tobacco in early and late age of initiation of smoking tobacco by different background characteristics. The respondents initiated in smoking tobacco in early age (3 per cent) and late age (8 per cent) were less likely in the urban area as compared with their counterpart in rural area. The respondents were more likely to initiate smoking tobacco at the age of ≥65 years in either early age (1.14 times) or late age (8.82 times) as compared with the reference category. Those respondents having education were significantly less likely in both early age and late age as compared with without formal education group. Therefore, respondents in the North-east region were significantly 1.14 times more likely as compared with the northern region to started smoking tobacco at an early age but less likely (17 per cent) in a late age at initiation of smoking tobacco.

Table 3 exhibits the prevalence and differential of early and late age at initiation of smokeless tobacco by different background characteristics. The prevalence of early age at initiation of smokeless tobacco is significantly lower as compared with late age. It accounts for 8.7 per cent and 12.1 per cent respectively. Nevertheless, the initiation of smokeless tobacco in early and late age is higher (10.2 percent and 13.4 per cent respectively) in the rural area as compared with the urban area (5.2 percent and 9.1 per cent respectively) which was evident with a study done by Rawat et al. (2016). Smokeless tobacco consumption (?) for both late and early ages was remarkably higher among respondents without formal schooling (11.1 percent and 16.5 per cent) and less in respondents having primary but less than secondary education (12.5 percent and 14.4 per cent).

Table 3. Prevalence of smokeless tobacco consumption initiation in early and late age by selected background characteristics in India, 2009-10

Background characteristics	Age at initiation of smokeless tobacco consumption			
	Early		Late	
	%	N	%	N
Place of residence				
Rural	10.2	3566	13.4	5137
Urban	5.2	1364	9.1	2375
Sex				
Male	11.1	3043	15.7	4757
Female	6.2	1887	8.3	2755
Age group (years)				
15-24	8.9	969	2.8	318
25-44	9.2	2675	14.1	4055
45-54	7.5	633	17.1	1442
55-64	7.6	348	20.0	900
65 and above	8.0	305	20.9	797
Education level				
No formal schooling	11.1	1851	16.5	2666
Less than primary	12.5	856	14.4	1161
Primary but less than secondary	9.0	1474	11.0	2149
Secondary and above	11.1	1851	16.5	2666
Occupation				
Govt. & non Govt. employed	12.0	1493	15.1	2119
Self-employed	11.6	1880	17.6	3037
Student	2.9	162	0.6	48
Homemaker	5.3	1053	8.3	1722
Retired and unemployed	9.9	335	15.7	564
National region				
North	2.1	311	3.8	571
Central	10.5	1083	13.9	1532
East	13.3	1331	16.7	1750
North-east	9.0	1250	11.8	1905
West	8.6	649	12.8	1063
South	3.3	306	6.8	691
India	8.7	4930	12.1	7512

Education has a direct effect on control tobacco use. Furthermore, respondents belong to the central and eastern regions have higher initiation of smokeless tobacco in the early age (10.5 per cent and 13.3 per cent respectively) and also in late age (13.9 per cent and 16.7 per cent respectively). This is also as per the study of Rawat (2014) and Rawat et al. (2016).

Table 4. Logistic regression analysis of early and late age at initiation of smokeless tobacco consumption by selected background characteristics in India, 2009-10

Background characteristics	Age at initiation of smokeless tobacco consumption	
	Early	Late
	ORs(L-U)	ORs(L-U)
Place of residence		
Rural®		
Urban	0.79***(0.74-0.85)	0.84***(0.80-0.89)
Sex		
Male®		
Female	0.63***(0.58-0.69)	0.60***(0.56-0.65)
Age (years)		
15-24®		
25-44	0.74***(0.68-0.80)	3.87***(3.42-4.38)
45-54	1.51***(0.45-1.57)	4.52***(3.96-5.16)
55-64	0.86***(0.41-1.53)	5.03***(4.37-5.79)
65 and above	1.47***(0.40-1.54)	5.62***(4.86-6.51)
Education level		
No formal schooling®		
Less than primary	0.92*(0.84-1.01)	0.99 (0.92-1.07)
Primary but less than secondary	0.64***(0.59-0.69)	0.88***(0.83-0.94)
Secondary and above	0.28***(0.26-0.31)	0.56***(0.52-0.60)
Occupation		
Govt. & non-Govt. employed®		
Self-employed	0.82***(0.76-0.88)	0.98 (0.92-1.04)
Student	0.30***(0.25-0.36)	0.20***(0.15-0.28)
Homemaker	0.48***(0.44-0.54)	0.64***(0.59-0.70)
Retired and unemployed	0.80***(0.70-0.92)	0.79***(0.71-0.88)
National Region		
North®		
Central	4.03***(3.53-4.59)	3.84***(3.47-4.26)
East	5.65***(4.97-6.43)	4.80***(4.34-5.31)
North-east	3.41***(3.00-3.88)	3.18***(2.88-3.51)
West	3.10***(2.69-3.56)	2.90***(2.60-3.27)
South	1.09 (0.93-1.28)	1.37***(1.22-1.53)

Note: ®Reference category; statistically significant at $^*p < 0.10$, $^{**}p < 0.05$, $^{***}p < 0.01$.

Table 4 presents the result of logistic regression of early and late age at initiation of smokeless tobacco with selected background characteristics. The female respondents were significantly less likely to be initiated in smokeless tobacco in both early (21 per cent) and late (16 per cent) ages as compared with males. The result depicts that the respondents' age of ≥65 years at initiation of smokeless tobacco was significantly 5.62 times more likely as compared with the reference category, while the same result is also found in the age group of 55-64 years (Rawat et al. 2016). Respondents who were self-employed were 18 per cent less likely to be in the early age as compared with the reference category. Respondents belonging to the eastern and central regions were 5.65 and 4.03 times more likely to be in the early age at initiation of smokeless tobacco, while in the late age it was 4.80 and 3.84 times more likely as compared with the reference category respectively.

Discussion and Conclusion

The study attempts to explore the initiation of smoking and smokeless tobacco by age in the categories of early and late age. Besides, it examines the possible socioeconomic and household correlates that could affect the prevalence of this initiation. It reveals that there is a vast number of people suffering from diseases related to tobacco like cardiovascular diseases, cancer, cavity, etc. The risks of tobacco use are highest among those who start its use early and continue it for a long time or until the end of life (Morris et al. 2011; Henningfield 1995). Even though adults know well about tobacco-related health hazards, they continue to do so. Males use tobacco more than females in both early and late ages at initiation. People using tobacco for a long time have a significant risk of tobacco-related morbidity or health hazards. Earlier studies documented various health problems among tobacco users. The basic health problems can be categorized into cardiovascular diseases (CVDs), pulmonary diseases and cancer. However, in coming decades CVDs may be a leading cause of death (Morris et al. 2011). Both smoking and smokeless tobacco consumption in the central and eastern regions was highly initiated in early age respectively.

In the rural parts of these regions, the main reasons for the higher initiation in both ages might be easy availability of tobacco products and their low cost.

The factors like age, residence, occupation and education were significantly associated for both ages (early and late) of initiation. Education is an essential factor in removing the higher initiation of tobacco consumption because the students who have the secondary and above education were less initiated in both ages (early and late). Higher initiation of tobacco was found in backward states as people are unemployed. They moved around without work, consuming tobacco. The economic status of respondents is a key to control tobacco consumption. It is used in early age and hence the prevention programmes especially need to address the youth (Gupta and Ray 2002 and 2007). Furthermore, any kind of assistance may help to quit tobacco consumption for the uneducated, less educated and old age groups, particularly with emphasis on health hazards

According to the World Health Organization (2008), India is the second largest consumer of tobacco products in the world. The Government of India has various laws for reducing tobacco consumption and bringing greater awareness regarding the harmful effects of its consumption under the WHO Framework Convention on Tobacco Control (FCTC) (WHO 2008 and 2009). Under it smoking is completely banned in many public and work places such as healthcare, educational and government facilities as well as in public transport. Furthermore, advertising through many forms of mass media is prohibited, although tobacco companies still may advertise at the point of sale, subject to some restrictions. There are some restrictions on tobacco sponsorship and the publicity of such sponsorship (Raw et al. 2009). The Government should make more strong laws to control the use and sale of tobacco products, and their violation should mean punishment (Taylor and Bettcher 2000).

The Government a launched the National Tobacco Control Programme (NTCP) to restrain tobacco use. The Adult Tobacco Survey is an essential component of the country's comprehensive tobacco control programme and reflects an efficient and systematic surveillance mechanism to monitor the tobacco epidemic through a collection of baseline data and study of key tobacco control indicators. Many other laws are also enacted to promote awareness among the people about the harmful effect of tobacco consumption (Reddy and Gupta 2004). In spite of a large number of laws and programmes, why do the people not reduce tobacco consumption? This needs to be a concern of our policymakers and health department. The present study strongly recommends tobacco intervention policies that can be effective in achieving a smoke-free society. They include increase in the price of tobacco products, anti-smoking advertising by mass media, smoke-free policies, tobacco hazards curricula in schools, restrictions on tobacco marketing opportunities for the tobacco industry as well as social norms that lead to increased tobacco consumption, especially for youth. To raise more awareness about the harm of tobacco products among the population, catchy programmes at the local level with the involvement of a local leader are needed.

Greater tobacco consumption indicates that the health warning on tobacco packages and products needs to be made more effective in enhancing awareness regarding tobacco-related health hazards among the public. Community participation is essential for public awareness to get good results. Furthermore, active media (print, electronic or social) targeting specific groups to disseminate necessary information is required at the local level.

The health care providers need to be sensitized and trained for playing a proactive role for behavioural change of tobacco users in the society. Their activities may include primary motivation, enhancing knowledge of dangers of continuing tobacco use and benefits of quitting it. Given the prevalence of tobacco uses in the country, there should be a national effort to prevent any further increase in its consumption, especially among vulnerable groups in rural areas. Health professionals need to be sensitized and ask the victims about the habit of tobacco use and offer help to quit it. We require a strict policy for sellers who sell tobacco products to the children. There is a ban on the sale of tobacco products in public places and within 100 yards of educational institutions. Besides, mandatory display of pictorial health warnings on all tobacco product packages exists. The study concludes that community participation is indispensable for reducing tobacco consumption in all its forms.

REFERENCES

Bean, M. K., Mitchell, K. S., Speizer, I. S., Wilson, D. B., Smith, B. N., & Fries, E. A. (2008). Rural adolescent attitudes toward smoking and weight loss: relationship to smoking status. *Nicotine & tobacco research*, 10(2), 279-286.

Bhojani, U. M., Chander, S. J., & Devadasan, N. (2009). Tobacco use and related factors among pre-university students in a college in Bangalore, India. *National Medical Journal of India*, *22*(6), 294.

Centers for Disease Control and Prevention (CDC). (1998). Selected cigarette smoking initiation and quitting behaviors among high school students--United States, 1997. *MMWR. Morbidity and mortality weekly report*, *47*(19), 386.

Chaloupka, F. J., Pacula, R. L., Farrelly, M. C., Johnston, L. D., & O'Malley, P. M. (1999). *Do higher cigarette prices encourage youth to use marijuana?* (No. w6939). National Bureau of Economic Research.

DiFranza, J. R., Savageau, J. A., Fletcher, K., O'Loughlin, J., Pbert, L., Ockene, J. K., & Wood, C. (2007). Symptoms of tobacco dependence after brief intermittent use: the Development and Assessment of Nicotine Dependence in Youth–2 study. *Archives of pediatrics & adolescent medicine*, *161*(7), 704-710.

Dikshit, R. P., & Kanhere, S. (2000). Tobacco habits and risk of lung, oropharyngeal and oral cavity cancer: a population-based case-control study in Bhopal, India. *International Journal of epidemiology*, *29*(4), 609-614.

Doll, R., Peto, R., Boreham, J., & Sutherland, I. (2004). Mortality in relation to smoking: 50 years' observations on male British doctors. *Bmj*, *328*(7455), 1519.

Eaton, D. K., Kann, L., Kinchen, S., Shanklin, S., Ross, J., Hawkins, J., & Lim, C. (2010). Youth risk behavior surveillance-United States, 2009. *MMWR Surveill Summ*, *59*(5), 1-142.

Gupta, P. C. (2006). Tobacco control in India. *Indian Journal of Medical Research*, *123*(5), 579.

Gupta, P. C., & RAY, C. S. (2002). Tobacco and youth in the South East Asian region. *Indian Journal of Cancer*, *39*(1), 5-34.

Gupta, P. C., & Ray, C. S. (2007). Tobacco, education & health. *Indian Journal of Medical Research*, *126*(4), 289.

Hegmann, K. T., Fraser, A. M., Keaney, R. P., Moser, S. E., Nilasena, D. S., Sedlars, M., & Lyon, J. L. (1993). The effect of age at smoking initiation on lung cancer risk. *Epidemiology*, 444-448.

Henningfield, J. (1995). Symptoms of substance dependence associated with use of cigarettes, alcohol, and illicit drugs... *MMWR: Morbidity & Mortality Weekly Report*, *44*(44), 830-839.

International Institute for Population Sciences. (2007). *India National Family Health Survey (NFHS-3), 2005-06* (Vol. 1). International Institute for Population Sciences.

Jha, P., & Chaloupka, F. J. (2000). *Tobacco control in developing countries*. Oxford University Press.

Jha, P., Ranson, M. K., Nguyen, S. N., & Yach, D. (2002). Estimates of global and regional smoking prevalence in 1995, by age and sex. *American journal of public health*, *92*(6), 1002-1006.

Johnston, L. D., O'Malley, P. M., Bachman, J. G., & Schulenberg, J. E. (2010). *Monitoring the Future national results on adolescent drug use: Overview of key findings*, 2009.

Krishnamurthy, S., Ramaswamy, R., Trivedi, U., & Zachariah, V. (1997). Tobacco use in rural Indian children. *Indian pediatrics*, *34*(10), 923-927.

Kumar, P. M., Poorni, S., & Ramachandran, S. (2006). Tobacco use among school children in Chennai city, India. *Indian journal of cancer*, *43*(3), 127.

Kwamanga, D. H. O., Odhiambo, J. A., & Amukoye, E. I. (2003). Prevalence and risk factors of smoking among secondary school students in Nairobi. *East African medical journal*, *80*(4), 207-212.

Mackay, J., & Crofton, J. (1996). Tobacco and the developing world. *British Medical Bulletin*, *52*(1), 206-221.

Merrill, J. C., Fox, K. S., Lewis, S. R., & Pulver, G. E. (1994). Cigarettes, alcohol, marijuana: Gateways to illicit drug use. *New York: National Center on Addiction and Substance Abuse at Columbia University.*

Mohan, S., Sarma, P. S., & Thankappan, K. R. (2005). Access to pocket money and low educational performance predict tobacco use among adolescent boys in Kerala, India. *Preventive Medicine*, *41*(2), 685-692.

Morris, C. D., May, M. G., Devine, K., Smith, S., DeHay, T., & Mahalik, J. (2011). Multiple perspectives on tobacco use among youth with mental health disorders and addictions. *American Journal of Health Promotion*, *25*(5_suppl), S31-S37.

Neufeld, K. J., Peters, D. H., Rani, M., Bonu, S., & Brooner, R. K. (2005). Regular use of alcohol and tobacco in India and its association with age, gender, and poverty. *Drug and alcohol dependence*, *77*(3), 283-291.

Pednekar, M. S., & Gupta, P. C. (2004). Tobacco use among school students in Goa, India. *Indian journal of public health*, *48*(3), 147.

Raw, M., Regan, S., Rigotti, N. A., & McNeill, A. (2009). A survey of tobacco dependence treatment guidelines in 31 countries. *Addiction*, *104*(7), 1243-1250.

Rawat, R. (2014). Influence of education and occupation on smokeless tobacco use in EAG states and Assam, (Eds.) Ranjan, A., & Tiwari, A. *Mortality and Health*. MLC Foundation, Bhopal (MP).

Rawat, R., Gouda, J., & Shekhar, C. (2016). Smokeless tobacco use among adult males in India and selected states: Assessment of education and occupation linkages. *Journal of Human Behavior in the Social Environment*, *26*(2), 236-246.

Reddy, K. S., & Gupta, P. C. (2004). *Report on tobacco control in India* Ministry of Health and Family Welfare.

Reddy, K. S., Perry, C. L., Stigler, M. H., & Arora, M. (2005). Is a tobacco epidemic looming among young people in urban India. *Lancet*, *367*, 589-94.

Retherford, R. D., & Choe, M. K. (1993). *Statistical models for causal analysis* (pp. 119-150). New York: Wiley.

Riggs, N. R., Chou, C. P., Li, C., & Pentz, M. A. (2007). Adolescent to emerging adulthood smoking trajectories: when do smoking trajectories diverge, and do they predict early adulthood nicotine dependence?. *Nicotine & Tobacco Research*, *9*(11), 1147-1154.

Singh, A., & Ladusingh, L. (2014). Prevalence and determinants of tobacco use in India: Evidence from recent global adult tobacco survey data. *PloS one*, *9*(12), e114073.

Sinha, D. N. (2002). *Report on the results of the Global youth tobacco survey in Uttar Pradesh.*

Sinha, D. N., Gupta, P. C., Ray, C. S., & Singh, P. K. (2012). Prevalence of smokeless tobacco use among adults in WHO South-East Asia. *Indian journal of cancer*, *49*(4), 342.

Sinha, D. N., Reddy, K. S., Rahman, K., Warren, C. W., Jones, N. R., & Asma, S. (2006). Linking Global Youth Tobacco Survey (GYTS) data to the WHO framework convention on tobacco control: the case for India. *Indian journal of public health*, *50*(2), 76.

Taylor, A. L., & Bettcher, D. W. (2000). WHO Framework Convention on Tobacco Control: a global ''good''for public health. *Bulletin of the World Health Organization*, *78*, 920-929.

World Health Organization. (2008). Fresh and alive: Mpower, WHO report on the global tobacco epidemic, 2008. *World Health Organization.*

World Health Organization. (2009). *WHO framework convention on tobacco control.* Geneva: WHO.

INDEX

U

V

W

Y

Related Nova Publications

Ototoxicity: Signs, Symptoms and Treatment

Editor: Gregg Colon

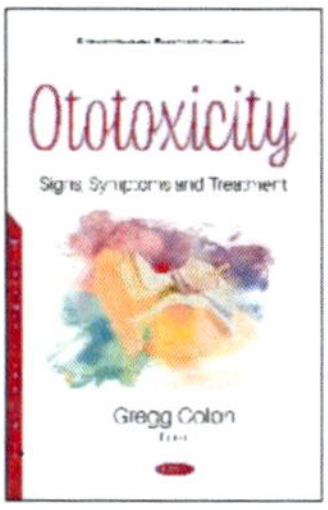

Series: Otolaryngology Research Advances

Book Description: This compilation focuses on ototoxicity, the adverse pharmacological reaction affecting the inner ear or auditory nerve, characterized by cochlear or vestibular dysfunction. Although ototoxic medications play an essential role in modern medicine, they can cause harm and lead to significant morbidity.

Softcover ISBN: 978-1-53616-396-4
Retail Price: $95

Substance Use Disorders in Adolescents and Young Adults: A Manual for Pediatric and Primary Care Clinicians. Second Edition

Editors: Donald E. Greydanus, MD, Gabriel Kaplan, MD, Dilip R. Patel, MD and Joav Merrick, MD, MMedSci, DMSc

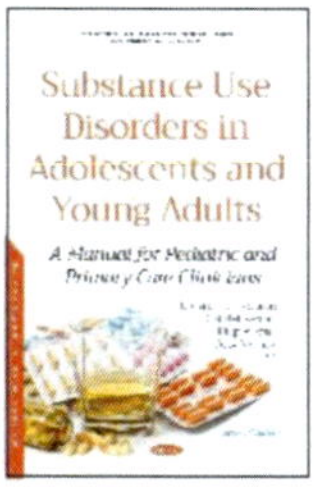

Series: Pediatrics, Child and Adolescent Health

Book Description: This updated and revised second edition on substance abuse in adolescents and young adults provides information on this global public health topic. We cover a wide variety of subjects within the paradigm of drug abuse and agree with the 21st century message of integrating substance abuse management with primary care services.

Hardcover ISBN: 978-1-53615-359-0
Retail Price: $230

To see a complete list of Nova publications, please visit our website at www.novapublishers.com